Little Miracles Everywhere

Little Miracles Everywhere

My Unorthodox Path to Holistic Veterinary Medicine

Marcie Fallek, DVM, CVA

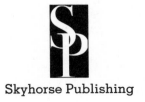

Skyhorse Publishing

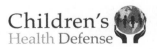

Copyright © 2024 by Marcie Fallek, DVM, CVA

Skyhorse Publishing books may be purchased in bulk at special discounts for sales promotion, corporate gifts, fund-raising, or educational purposes. Special editions can also be created to specifications. For details, contact the Special Sales Department, Skyhorse Publishing, 307 West 36th Street, 11th Floor, New York, NY 10018 or info@skyhorsepublishing.com.

Skyhorse® and Skyhorse Publishing® are registered trademarks of Skyhorse Publishing, Inc.®, a Delaware corporation.

Visit our website at www.skyhorsepublishing.com.

Please follow our publisher Tony Lyons on Instagram @tonylyonsisuncertain

10 9 8 7 6 5 4 3

Library of Congress Cataloging-in-Publication Data is available on file.

Cover design by David Ter-Avanesyan
Cover image provided by Marcie Fallek

Print ISBN: 978-1-5107-8202-0
Ebook ISBN: 978-1-5107-8251-8

Printed in the United States of America

For my grandmother, Betty Schreiber,
whose love lit my life, and whose faith in me never wavered.

Contents

Prologue ix

Chapter 1: Divine Intervention Needed 1
Chapter 2: Seeking Creature Comforts 6
Chapter 3: A Rod and a Promise 11
Chapter 4: A Divine Coincidence 16
Chapter 5: From Butcher to Binger 20
Chapter 6: Ten Weeks to Chutzpa 25
Chapter 7: Partners, *Pallini*, and *Prosciutto* 30
Chapter 8: The Doctor Makes a Deal 38
Chapter 9: An Alternate Reality 42
Chapter 10: Wait, More Tests? 45
Chapter 11: Cows Kick Sideways 49
Chapter 12: DIY Doctoring 55
Chapter 13: Castration to CATastrophy 61
Chapter 14: Chop Chops and Veal Chops 66
Chapter 15: Bovine, 'er Divine, Intervention 73
Chapter 16: Pass the Nutmeg 79
Chapter 17: From Shabby to Chic 82
Chapter 18: "Mr. Newman in Room One" 87
Chapter 19: Two Hearts Opened 93
Chapter 20: Just Like the Ashram 99
Chapter 21: A Friend and a Firing 103
Chapter 22: "Kill the Kittens" 108
Chapter 23: Like Brothers I Never Had 112
Chapter 24: Diagnostics and Detective Work 118
Chapter 25: A Crash Splits the Air 122

Chapter 26: A New Business   126

Chapter 27: Get Used to It Now   131

Chapter 28: A Punch in the Gut   135

Chapter 29: A Curious Cause   140

Chapter 30: A New Path Appears   145

Chapter 31: Ten Bucks an Hour   151

Chapter 32: "This Will Never Break"   155

Chapter 33: A New Way to Heal   159

Chapter 34: A Growing List of Miracles   164

Chapter 35: Parting Ways   172

Chapter 36: Countdown to Aspen   178

Chapter 37: Cause and Effect   183

Chapter 38: Roadkill for Dinner   188

Chapter 39: Risks vs. Benefits   192

Chapter 40: From God's Mouth   198

Chapter 41: A Deadly Prognosis   203

Chapter 42: A String of Successes   210

Chapter 43: A Death and Resurrection   217

Chapter 44: A Thanksgiving Miracle   222

Chapter 45: Dreams of Manhattan   227

Chapter 46: The Right Wrong Number   232

Epilogue   235

Acknowledgments   246

Prologue

A middle-aged brunette entered my office holding a three-pound skeleton strapped to a wooden plank. I could barely make out the creature. I directed the woman toward the exam table, on which she tenderly placed the planked animal. A cat. Each gasped breath from the creature seemed to be its last.

I had hoped the opening day of my new Greenwich Village clinic in New York City would be easy. From a long list of pet owners calling for help, I had returned Andrea's call first. She had told me that her fourteen-year-old cat was in kidney failure, something I'd had good success treating in the past. I'd thought maybe I could add a few more years to this animal's life. Now I hoped he'd make it through the appointment.

"So, tell me what's going on with Archie," I managed. "You told me he had chronic kidney failure. Is there more to the story?"

"Well, he also has lung cancer," Andrea admitted. "I was afraid if I told you how bad he was, you wouldn't see me."

She was probably right.

I placed my hand on her shoulder. "Andrea, your cat is much sicker than I'd thought. I'm afraid he's beyond my help." I had witnessed so many miraculous healings with holistic medicine that I'd rarely had to recommend euthanasia, but I could not, in good conscience, encourage this woman to pursue any treatment, including my own. Accepting her money wouldn't feel ethical.

"He wants to live; I know he does. Please try!" she pleaded. She told me she'd taken him out of a sewer in Manhattan when he was a kitten. "He fought and struggled his whole life to survive. He's been there for me in every crisis of my life. Now I need to be here for him. I owe it to him."

Andrea was crying now, and my heart melted. I gave her a hug. Despite my misgivings about being able to help this cat, how could I say no?

"OK. I'll try."

I pulled a chair to one side of the table for Andrea and rolled my chair to the other side. I inserted a fresh treatment record into my clipboard. "Let's start from the beginning."

Archie had been diagnosed with advanced kidney failure and had defied his veterinarians' predictions of imminent death for the past four years. His latest renal ultrasound showed that his kidneys were "incompatible with life," she said. Despite that report, with Andrea's daily administration of subcutaneous fluids, the cat had thrived. That is, until Andrea went on a two-week vacation, leaving Archie with his usual cat-sitter.

When Andrea returned, she found Archie in the condition that I now observed: a barely breathing bag of skin and bones. Andrea had rushed the cat to her regular vet, who diagnosed heart failure. But heart drugs, he told her, would only exacerbate the kidney failure. The only option was euthanasia, the vet said.

Andrea ignored the doctor and went straight to Animal Medical Center (AMC), Manhattan's most prestigious veterinary hospital. Several tests later, the specialists diagnosed advanced lung cancer (in addition to the kidney failure). Heart failure was a misdiagnosis, they said. They drained fluid from the cat's chest cavity to ease his labored breathing and recommended euthanasia.

Andrea had refused and brought the cat home. She returned to the AMC for additional chest taps, but Archie remained subdued and wouldn't eat. After the third visit, the veterinarians at the AMC told Andrea another tap would be too dangerous. They refused to treat the cat anymore.

That's when she called me.

Over the years, I accumulated many tools for my holistic toolbox. I specialize in acupuncture and classical homeopathy, two powerful energy healing modalities. But Archie's condition was precarious, and even holistic treatment carried risk for an animal in this state. I'd heard one report of acupuncture healing a case of cancer, but our professors at the International Veterinary Acupuncture Society (IVAS) had warned that treating an animal with cancer could accelerate a malignancy. Homeopathy is safe and gentle, even for cancer, but when an animal is close to death all bets are off.

While Andrea stroked Archie, I asked dozens of questions, inputting the answers into the homeopathic program on my computer, which helped narrow down the thousands of available remedies into the most appropriate for this poor creature.

Arsenicum album. According to the program, this remedy seemed most likely to help Archie. Through experience, I knew it was also one of two remedies that helps an animal on the brink of death to transition peacefully. That was not my intention here, so I searched for an alternative. But *Arsenicum album* was the only remedy that fit the case.

I told Andrea to administer one drop a day to the cat, the lowest possible dose, to keep a daily log, and to call me in two days.

She didn't call. I suspected the worst.

Two weeks later, Andrea called.

"Is Archie OK?" I blurted out.

"He's much better!"

The cat was alive? *Thank you, God.* "What are you seeing?" I said.

"His breathing is better, he's more alert, and he's eating on his own."

Astonishing. But the cat was not out of the woods. "Increase the *Arsenicum* to one drop twice a day. If Archie worsens, stop the remedy and call me. If he improves, please call me in two weeks."

Two weeks later, Andrea telephoned with a concern. "He's peeing tons of urine!"

Increased urination could mean the kidney disease had worsened. "Is he vomiting?"

"No, he's eating normally. In fact, he's feeling really good."

"Are his stools small, hard, and dry, like before?" A sign of dehydration. She told me they looked normal.

"How is his breathing?"

"Much better. Actually, it seems normal."

Archie wasn't showing any signs of kidney disease, and he hadn't had another chest tap. It seemed crazy, but I surmised that his body was purging the fluid in his lungs through his kidneys. I'd never seen that before, but it was the only logical explanation.

I had to see for myself. I asked Andrea to bring Archie back for a recheck the following week.

On Saturday, she toted her cat in a carrier. No more plank. Archie looked like a healthy, young cat. His coat was shiny, he had regained all his weight, and he had a sparkle in his eyes. I couldn't believe the transformation.

Archie was *thriving* despite his lung cancer and kidney failure.

Andrea's love and dedication, and Archie's determination to live, taught me this: the impossible *can* become possible.

Chapter 1

Divine Intervention Needed

A blast of hot, dank air hit me as soon as I stepped off the plane in Bombay. It must have been 100 degrees, even though it was after midnight. Beyond exhausted, I trailed fifty-nine other pilgrims, as Raimondo, our group leader from Italy, shepherded us toward our waiting luggage. We wound our way through throngs of pushing and shoving Indians toward the taxi stand.

I was a twenty-seven-year-old Jewish New Yorker studying veterinary medicine in Italy at the Università di Bologna. I'd made this journey from Italy during Christmas break for the same reasons the others had: we'd been told that God lived in India. Finding God had been on my to-do list for as long as I could remember.

Plus, I'd need Divine intervention to pass my veterinary exams.

Veterinary school in Bologna was a five-year program—in Italian—and students needed to pass fifty-one oral exams to graduate. I'd passed only fourteen in four years. In other words, I had thirty-eight to go. In one year. Theoretically, anyway. Like with most things Italian, rules could be broken. Students were allowed *twenty years* to get through. If you exceeded that, you'd have to start all over again.

About 60 percent of Americans and 80 percent of Italians flunked out. This terrified me. I'd never failed an exam in my life. I needed help.

I crowded into a taxi with four strangers. Through sleep-deprived eyes, I spied thousands of lifeless lumps littering the ground outside the airport. "They're people!" someone muttered.

I spent a sleepless night at a no-star hotel in Bombay and the next morning squeezed into another dilapidated taxi with four more strangers for the second leg of our journey. The driver piled our luggage high onto the roof and tied it down with rope, then slid behind the wheel and sped off through vehicular anarchy, bumping and bouncing along what was generously called a road. I kept a wary eye out the rear window for my green plaid suitcase.

What had I gotten myself into? I prayed for safe passage and reviewed my motivations: Find God and finish vet school.

My miserable childhood had launched this journey to find God. At seven years old, as I lay in bed curled in a tight ball, hugging myself and sobbing, I felt there had to be something more to life than the anger that filled our home. I cried out to a God I wasn't sure was there.

In college, I'd majored in philosophy. *Why am I here?* Why were any of us here? Time and again I wondered: how could I live a purposeful life that also made me happy? I knew one thing: animals made me happy.

In India, I stared out the window as a kaleidoscope of unfamiliar sights, sounds, and smells assaulted my senses. Human skeletons in loincloths pulled or pedaled rickshaws. Beautiful, floppy-eared white oxen strained heroically, lugging heavy wooden carts. Skinny men controlled them using thick, painful-looking rope shoved through the animals' nostrils. The sight pierced my heart. Mildew mixed with incense, manure, and pungent Indian spices smelled not unpleasant. Indians, some with goats tethered to short leashes, cooked on open fires along the side of the road. I turned away, hoping the animals wouldn't end up in the pots.

My heart soared when I noticed some charming Brahman cattle meandering through the traffic, their necks draped with flowers and golden bells tinkling on their horns. I loved seeing them free and happy.

When we stopped at a red light, adolescent boys with broad smiles shoved their leprosy-eaten arms into our taxi windows. I recoiled. Babu, our driver, waved them away. I watched them move undeterred to the next car.

We took a short flight to Bangalore and then boarded a large tour bus for a seven-hour ride to the ashram, which a fellow pilgrim had described as five minutes from the Stone Age. I peered out the window from my seat right behind Mohammed, the driver. Alone, yet not alone, my preferred state of being. Brush and boulders dotted the barren terrain. Herds of goats and sheep blocked our path on the dusty, narrow road. We waited while young, sandal-clad shepherds drove them out of our way with curved wooden canes. This felt like a scene straight out of the Bible.

Halfway to the ashram, Mohammed pulled over to the side of the road for a pee stop. I stepped out cautiously and looked around for toilets. A stocky, middle-aged brunette named Chiara noticed my confusion and pointed to a rock. "Pick a big one. But watch out for cobras. Those red mounds are cobra nests."

After three more hours of dust and rock and goats, just as I began to nod off, pink archways decorated with sculptures of angels and peacocks and other creatures sprouted up from the colorless terrain. We passed through an archway bordered by lotus flowers and symbols of various religions. Pastel-colored buildings lined the widening dirt road.

Mohammed turned to us. "We're almost there."

My heart pounded. This was where Sai Baba, an avatar or incarnation of God, supposedly lived, in *Prashanthi Nilayam,* or Abode of Highest Peace. I'd heard about Sai Baba during my first year of vet school. I'd befriended an Italian kindergarten teacher who'd visited this ashram with a small group led by Antonio Craxi, the brother of the Italian prime minister. Her name was Anna, and she'd told me fantastical stories about this so-called miracle man. He'd materialized jewelry out of thin air, she said, returned sight to the blind, cured cancer with a powder—*vibhuti*—that he created with a mere wave of his hand. Anna even spoke about people raised from the dead. Sai Baba, she said, knew our past, present, and future, could manifest himself in many places at the same time, and could multiply food, just like Jesus.

Although I was Jewish, I'd always had a soft spot for Jesus. When I was little and our maid, Nellie, invited me to her Baptist church, I went. I loved the singing and appreciated the religious zeal, but, even at nine years old, I questioned the dogma: whoever didn't believe in Jesus would go to hell? I knew that if there was a God, he wouldn't send millions of faithful Jews, Muslims, Buddhists, Hindus, and the rest to hell, so I kept looking.

When I was ten, I walked with my grandma down Madison Avenue in Manhattan. I watched groups of other ten-year-old girls skipping down the street in their green plaid matching Catholic school uniforms and crisp white blouses. They looked like they were having a blast. They reminded me of Hayley Mills and her friends in *The Trouble with Angels*, a favorite movie of mine. But, dogma-wise, the Catholics sounded the same as the Baptists.

In high school, my friend Anne invited me to Kingdom Hall for Jehovah's Witness meetings. I warmed to their fellowship but didn't believe I'd die along with the other heathens in the coming Armageddon of 1984.

And try as I might, I couldn't find God during Friday night Shabbat services with my family at our reform Jewish synagogue. No one I met there even seemed to believe in God. Not my parents, not their friends, not my friends. I even had my doubts about the rabbi.

Like many Jewish New York liberals, I was a skeptic. But I've always had an open mind. Although I didn't think Jesus was God, if I'd been around two thousand years ago, I know I would have tried to make the trip to Jerusalem to see if the rumors were true. So, I had to do as much for Sai Baba. His teachings, which I'd read before the trip, resonated with what my inner voice whispered:

> There is only one religion; the religion of Love
> There is only one language; the language of the Heart
> There is only one caste; the caste of Humanity
> There is only one God; He is omnipresent.[1]

In other words, one God for all.

In my freshman year at Emory University in Atlanta, my Christian roommate had gifted me the book *Siddhartha*, which introduced me to Eastern Spirituality. That led me to Yogananda's *The Autobiography of a Yogi*. The author's experiences tugged at my soul. I knew I would get to India, the land of miracles, when the time was right.

---

1   Samuel H. Sandweiss, MD, *SAI BABA: The Holy Man . . . And The Psychiatrist* (San Diego, CA: Birth Day Publishing Company, 1975).

Our bus passed through a golden, wrought-iron gate into the ashram, and I felt like I'd entered another dimension. I spotted the temple, or *mandir*, to my left. It looked like a fancy double-decker wedding cake designed by Walt Disney, painted in the same pretty pastel colors as the archways and adorned with sculptures of swans, lions, elephants, and angels. Here, they told us, we would gather to pray, chant, and see Sai Baba during *Darshan*, the holiest part of the trip. Next to the mandir stood a tall, lotus-shaped cement pillar decorated with symbols of the world's major religions: the Om (Hindu), the Cross (Christian), the Star and Crescent (Muslim), the Buddhist Wheel (Buddhism), and Fire (Zoroastrianism, someone told me.)

I'd read about Sai Baba's teachings in Dr. Samuel Sandweiss's book, *The Holy Man and the Psychiatrist*. Dr. Sandweiss was Jewish, a skeptic, and a seeker, like me. In the 1970s, he'd traveled to India as a clinical psychiatrist to discredit Sai Baba. Instead, Sandweiss returned a changed man and a devotee.

But he'd already finished medical school. I still had thirty-eight exams to go.

Chapter 2

Seeking Creature Comforts

Man-pedaled rickshaws took us to our assigned rooms. I dragged my luggage up two flights of stairs and down a long, outdoor, verandah-like hallway. Someone opened the door to our room, and I found myself staring into an empty twenty-by-twenty-foot cement-floored room to be shared by all eight women in my group. A single snore by any of them, and I knew my sleeping would be over.

You can take the New Yorker out of New York. But take New York out of the New Yorker? Not so much. I raced to drop my bag alongside a wall to claim a six-by-three-foot piece of real estate. Then I looked around. A sad-eyed, middle-aged woman, whom I'd noticed alone in the bus, had begun to set up a makeshift altar. Despite her full-length mink coat, I felt drawn to her. A lonely, kindred spirit? Overcoming my shyness, I stuck out my hand and introduced myself.

"*Mi chiama* Adriana," she said in Italian, telling me her name. She placed what looked like a crystal necklace around a framed photo of Sai Baba.

"That's beautiful," I said. "What is it?"

"It's Pope John XXIII's crucifix. My husband was with the pope when he died. Papa Giovanni wanted my husband to have it."

The pope?! I eyed the beads with reverence. I didn't know much about popes, but I believed this guy was one of the good ones. Suddenly aware of my frayed and worn-out Indian style dress, the one I'd kept from my hippy days at college, I said "What does your husband do?"

"He's an MP (member of parliament). He's ultra-conservative. I'm not. Our marriage is not the happiest," she confided. "For ten years he wouldn't let me come here. I don't know why he changed his mind. Maybe he has a girlfriend now." She turned back toward the altar and adjusted the rosary.

I felt for her and was touched by the confidence she'd shared. I tried to give her her space (what little there was, anyway).

Chiara walked over. She'd told me at the pit stop that this was her second trip to the ashram, so she knew the ropes. She invited me to walk with her to the village of Puttaparthi to buy mattresses and a plastic pail and cup for washing up.

I followed Chiara down the stairs and retraced our route to the ashram gate. Once outside Ganesha Gate, I froze. Shrouded figures with gaping black holes in their faces sat on the opposite curb, arms outstretched. More leprosy.

I turned to my right, where a legless boy propelled himself by his arms on a crude wooden pallet. Horrified, I looked to my left and saw half a dozen grimy, barefoot girls, no older than eight, supporting tiny infants on their hips with one arm, while the other reached toward us, begging for change.

"Ignore them!" Chiara commanded. "Baba says we can give food, but not money. Hurry up or we'll be late for the group meeting." I stifled my well-fed guilt and followed Chiara as she picked her way through garbage to an open-air stall where a scrawny Indian man pedaled an old-fashioned sewing machine. We were sari-shopping, apparently. The man looked up with a toothless grin and waved us into the dark bowels of the shop. I followed Chiara's lead and removed my shoes before I entered. How strange to be so fastidious surrounded by all the filth.

The shopkeeper loaded dozens of neatly folded, multicolored saris wrapped in stiff plastic on the narrow countertop. Most were paisley-patterned geometrical shapes that seemed downright dowdy. I managed to find a beautiful sheer powder blue one with delicate pink roses. The tailor measured me for a matching blouse and petticoat that I'd pick up later.

As we made our way through piles of cow dung to the next shop, a motorized rickshaw crossed our path. On the rear window was plastered a decal: "If God seems far away, guess who moved." India's spiritual wealth, juxtaposed with unfathomable material poverty.

I followed Chiara into a stall filled with piles of two-inch thick mattresses and other home goods. "Get two mattresses," Chiara advised, "it'll be more comfortable, and they're only ten rupees (one dollar)." At the third shop we purchased a plastic bucket and cup for "washing up."

Chiara laughed at my expression. "At least our room has running water," she said, referring to the single waist-high spigot of cold water and hole in the floor in our "bathroom." We'd have to fill the bucket with water, then dip the cup into the bucket and pour it over ourselves many times. "We are lucky to have a room," she continued. "Most people stay in a shed." The sheds housed up to two hundred people each and had no indoor plumbing. Those pilgrims drew water from a single outdoor well to wash and used outhouses in lieu of toilets.

Despite Chiara's assurances of our good fortune, and my silent pep talk about how I'd come to India to meet God and not to have a five-star vacation, I dreaded what lay ahead. I suffered from terrible insomnia and had an overactive bladder.

On the way to the stores, I took note of a "Hotel" sign hanging over a small thatched hut and made a mental note to check it out later.

Back inside the ashram, I read some of Baba's phrases painted on cement slabs lining the dirt road to the mandir:

"Work Is Worship."
"Hands that Help Are Holier than Lips that Pray."
"Service to Man Is Service to God."
"Love All, Serve All."

I took this to mean animals as well!

We passed ancient-looking, permanently bent-over women in saris, sweeping the immaculate dirt path with bundles of twig-like grasses tied together. They looked like characters out of Grimm's Fairy Tales.

We dumped our stuff in our room and raced to the orientation room. We seated ourselves on the floor behind the other women. The men sat on the other side, separated from us by a wide aisle. Raimondo spelled out our schedule, along with the rules and regulations.

"This is a spiritual journey," Raimondo counseled. "We are not here to make friends or sightsee. Remember, it is in the silence that you find God." Smoking, alcohol, drugs, and meat, as well as fraternizing with the opposite sex, were prohibited on ashram grounds. He eyed some fellow Italian pilgrims. "This also means outside the ashram. No leaning on the ashram wall smoking with your arm around your girlfriend."

After the meeting, Chiara invited me to the canteen for dinner, but I declined so I could check out that hotel. I mustered the courage to exit Ganesha Gate once again and hurried toward the hotel.

An Indian man waved. "Hotel?" he called.

I nodded. "How much?"

"Twenty rupees."

Two dollars. I peered into a cave-like hut. No windows and a dirt floor. Still, it would be all mine. I hesitated, weighing my options.

"You have to watch out for tarantulas," he cautioned.

That did it. I dashed back to the ashram.

The others were still at dinner while I unpacked, ate some crackers and peanut butter I'd brought from Bologna, and then slipped on my cotton nightgown. I made up my double layer bed with sheets I'd brought from Italy and some cotton blankets I'd bought with the mattress. I inserted my Calmor wax ear plugs, wrapped my head in my Brookstone eyeshades, slid under the covers, and waited for the other women to return.

By eight, they arrived. I pretended to sleep. Shortly after the lights went out, at 9 p.m., the cacophony of snoring began.

I lay there for about half an hour, searching for a solution.

Got it! I dragged my mattresses outside to the verandah, where the cool silence soothed my nerves. I lay down, covered my head with my blanket, and prayed for sleep to someone I hoped was listening.

A few miserable, sleepless hours later, somebody's alarm blared: the 3:30 a.m. wakeup call. I poked my head out of the covers and discovered three large, bald creatures with pointy faces and open sores huddled on the edge of my blanket. They looked like oversized rats. And contagious. I screamed.

They fled.

Only then did I realize that they were dogs. I'd never in my life seen canines that looked that pitiful. Compassion swelled in me, along with deep shame. These creatures had only wanted my company and warmth. The very creatures I'd hoped to help someday, if my quest to become a veterinarian ever materialized.

Chapter 3

A Rod and a Promise

OM-ing and meditation started at 4 a.m. sharp, and I was exhausted. It had been seventy-two hours since I'd gotten any sleep. With a sigh, I dragged my mattresses back inside, threw on some clothes, and stumbled after my group in the darkness to the mandir.

I filed into the inner sanctuary with the others and looked around in wonder. The predawn darkness, lit only by candles on the altar, along with the mystical animal sculptures and life-sized statues and portraits of the many incarnations of God gracing the dais, infused the room with an otherworldly holiness.

I sat on the cold marble floor, clutching my crossed knees into my chest and squeezed in among dozens of sari-d women. A wide aisle covered with red carpet separated us from the men, all dressed in white pajamas.

A sense of expectation filled the room. Rolling waves of Oms reverberated from and through the crowd—*Omkar*, repeating Om twenty-one times. Raimondo had told us about this at orientation. My anxiety melted as I merged with the waves. But me and my ADD self couldn't stop thinking of the lepers and begging children. And those dogs. I felt awful that I'd scared them off. I hoped I could make it up to them.

I began to cough uncontrollably. I tensed, expecting to be yelled at like in a New York movie theater, or by my mother or sister when I screwed something up. Instead, someone rubbed my back. I flinched. I hated to be touched, even in a nice way, even when my grandma held my hand. A sari'd arm passed me a hard candy; the kindness took me by surprise.

Half an hour later, we exited the sanctuary into the still-dark morning. Under a star-studded sky, I followed the others as they circled the mandir, chanting devotional songs, *bhajans*.

Then we scattered, back to the room for a bucket bath and to dress in our saris for Darshan. For the life of me, I couldn't figure out how to wrap the long piece of cloth around me to look anything like a sari. All that folding and pleating and pinning. Chiara took pity and helped.

"You look beautiful in a sari," my new friend Adriana exclaimed. "It suits you; you are so tall and slim. And with your curly blonde hair you look like an angel!"

It may have suited me, but I felt like a mummy swathed in plastic wrap. I shuffled off to the canteen with the others. I needed caffeine and something to eat.

I took my place at the end of the women's queue, grabbed a tray from the large stack, and made my way down the serving line. I nodded "yes" as a *seva* (volunteer) doled out some kind of porridge from a huge metal cauldron onto a stainless-steel plate. The next seva handed me a piece of flatbread. I took half a dozen tiny metal cups filled with a milky-looking hot drink from the end of the table, hoping they contained caffeine.

I carried my tray to one of the long cement tables that filled the room and slid onto its attached bench next to other devotees. I glanced at my neighbors. How was I supposed to eat hot porridge without utensils? They used their fingers. When in Rome . . .

Spicy farina and chai tea. Delicious!

On my way to the temple, my mind drifted back to the dogs. Mange! That's why they were bald! They'd scratched all their hair off, leaving only open sores. There'd been no mention of that in vet school at the University of Bologna, which was founded in 1088 and probably hadn't changed much over the millennia. It still focused on farm and draught animals, like cows and horses and pigs, and considered dogs and cats superfluous. But thanks to the veterinarians at our family dog's hospital where I'd volunteered after college, I knew that mange was treatable. Four weekly lime *Sulphur* dips—if I recalled correctly. That, plus food, and they'd be normal dogs—like Nika, the sheltie mix I'd left at home with my parents when I took off for Bologna.

Enough with the daydreaming. I checked my watch. It was time to meet God.

I hurried toward the mandir and spotted my group already queued up outside.

A severe-faced seva, identified by a blue neck scarf, held up her hand, palm toward New Yorker me. *Slow down.* We filed in one by one. Sevas stood like sentries at both ends of each row, directing us toward seating. One after the other, various sevas shooed me forward until I reached the first row (!), a not-so-small miracle in this crowd of twenty thousand people. I felt as if a fairy godmother had waved a magic wand over my head.

I sat cross-legged in the sand, struck by my luck.

From the corner of my eye, I spotted a blond-haired, blue-eyed woman and a girl around three years old, sitting diagonally behind me. They appeared to be Scandinavian, with their tall Nordic beauty. The girl, apparently the woman's daughter, was picture perfect, like a child movie star, except for a huge red tumor that hung from her neck. I felt sick to my stomach at the sight, but their faces glowed. I imagined the mom hoped Baba would heal her daughter.

Women with frozen limbs, twisted and contorted into all sorts of impossible shapes, lay in wheelchairs parked along the retaining wall of the temple. Despite their infirmities, the women's faces radiated devotion.

I wanted what they seemed to have. Faith? Something to replace my constant anxiety. I had to pass thirty-eight more exams but compared to them, I should be living in a constant state of gratitude.

A small army of children, immaculately dressed in white, marched in from behind the mandir and took their places on the verandah, little five-year-olds in front, sloping upward to the tallest teenagers in back.

The unrelenting Indian sun beat down on us as we waited for Baba. An Indian girl on my right wrote and rewrote the Hindu symbol for Om in meticulous script into a small, lined notebook. An old woman to my left muttered prayers from a booklet she held in her lap. Some Indians fanned themselves with pieces of paper, others with mini battery-powered fans.

Suddenly, soft instrumental music filled the air. Everyone came to attention, with their palms pressed together in the Namaste pose, fingers pointing upward and thumbs to chest. I copied them, my gaze following theirs, as heads turned toward the mandir door.

The door opened and a small brown man with a large Afro glided across the sand toward us. Sai Baba. He seemed to float—his feet hidden under the hem of his full-length orange robe. He paused and scanned the crowd. Then he lifted his gaze, focusing on some point above and beyond us.

I stared, unsure what to think.

He made his way along the edge of the crowd, starting on the women's side. As he approached, many rose to their knees, hands still pressed together, attempting to get his attention. Baba ignored some and spoke to others. Several reached out to touch his feet. If someone was too pushy, Baba glowered.

Some held out letters for him to collect, others, infants to bless. After he'd passed, devotees gathered the grains of sand that he'd tread on, folding them carefully into pieces of paper torn from books or notebooks, which to me seemed over the top.

Suddenly Baba turned toward me and looked straight into my eyes.

I felt like he was staring into my soul, like somehow, he knew everything about me—my struggles with my family, my struggles with my studies. He knew how hard I tried, with everything. To be good, to do the right thing. At that moment it was as if nothing else mattered except what God thought of me. The real me.

I hoped I'd lived up to his expectations.

And then, without a word, Baba moved on, making his way slowly toward the men's section.

Baba's gaze somehow triggered something deep inside, because a truth hit me like a lightning bolt: I, alone, was responsible for my life—my every thought, my every action. There *was* a God who saw, knew, and understood. I determined not to let Him down.

I needed time alone. I decided to skip the food line and instead took a walk. I found a bakery across from the canteen, a real bakery with real loaves of bread, my favorite food. Wrapped in old newspaper, a loaf of whole-wheat cost only two rupees (twenty cents). I bought one, ate half, and dropped the rest in my new Indian hand-embroidered cotton shoulder bag and continued exploring.

Rounding the corner past the mandir, I spotted an emaciated dog hiding in the brush. I took out the bread from my bag and approached cautiously, not wanting to scare him off. A seva intercepted us, brandishing a metal club. The dog howled and bolted before the steel rod could reach him. The guard shot me a grin, convinced he'd protected me from some awful fate. Given the cultural divide, I didn't feel it my place to confront him. But the rod crushed my spirit.

When I saw the guard raise his club outside the mandir, I *was* that dog. My mind flashed back to when I was seven years old. I was locked in the bathroom, lying on the floor. Soul-wracking sobs arose from a place so deep within me that I felt they possessed my body. I *was* the screaming. I *was* the pain. My mother had gotten me a few times with the belt in my bedroom. For the first time ever, I slapped her back. Enraged, her beating became even more ferocious. "Don't you ever hit me!" she roared.

I ran away from the mandir and the guard and searched for the dog, but I couldn't find him. Dejected, I sat on the dirt road under the shade of a tree. Across the path I spotted a cement slab hand-painted with the Sai Baba dictum: "God Is Love." My heart felt heavy as I considered the lot of most animals the world over: helpless victims. They endured chains, whips, shelters, zoos, slaughterhouses. They lived or died according to our whims.

I stared at those words and vowed there and then to finish vet school, so I could help and heal and love as many animals as I could in India and beyond.

Chapter 4

A Divine Coincidence

As I walked back to our room, I spotted Adriana kneeling in front of a large blackboard, writing something into a tiny notebook. With her matching gold pen, she was copying Sai Baba's "Thought of the Day." She looked up at me, tore the sheet of paper from the notebook, and stuffed it in her purse. I peered at the notebook, the word "Cartier" embossed in gold lettering on the red leather. I'd never seen such a fine notebook and pen set. "You're ruining Cartier!" I cried.

Adriana turned to me with a wry smile. "Cartier ruined me," she said. Her sorrowful eyes spoke volumes.

I continued alone, back to the room.

Night Two: I dragged my mattresses out on the verandah again. I couldn't sleep as my mind raced, reliving the day: People kissing the feet of some guy they claimed was God. Mythical statues. Hypnotic chanting. Candles in the dark. Incense. Men in loincloths. Witches with brooms. The rainbow-colored Walt Disney temple. I'd even met a chubby young Indian girl who told me she'd died. (Actually, that she'd been dead for three whole days!) She said Baba had resurrected her. I took her picture.

I am a sober and serious person. The only drug I ever tried was my mom's diet pills, which she gave me at fifteen when she said I should lose a few pounds. But at the ashram, I felt like I was on an LSD trip.

The alarm sounded promptly at 3:30 a.m. No dogs this time, and still no sleep. Somehow, I made it to the mandir. Baba stood right in front of me during Darshan and spoke to the woman on my right. The woman to my left nudged me. "Kiss his feet! It will bring you great spiritual boons." Really? Too weird. She nudged me again. *What if he really was God?* Just in case, I lowered my head and touched my lips to his feet. Their softness startled me.

Fast forward to day five. Baba called our Italian group for an interview—a private audience—sought by all, including me.

Raimondo had spelled out the protocol for what to do if Baba called. Enter silently, don't push. I couldn't help myself, being a typical New Yorker, as soon as I entered the interview room and spotted a single, red, satin-covered chair no doubt meant for Baba, I wriggled my way to the front and plopped down on the floor a foot from the chair. Ring-side seat! The other fifty-nine devotees crammed in behind me.

Baba entered, closed the door behind him, and took his seat on the chair. The room and its occupants disappeared as I stared transfixed at the little man with the big afro, the man whom millions called God.

Baba smiled and welcomed us in English to what he called our "spiritual home." Then in Italian (he spoke Italian!), he joked that our interview was *divino* (divine), not *di vino* (of wine).

Baba held up his handkerchief. "What is this?"

Someone called out, "handkerchief."

"Cloth. Cloth is made of thread," Baba said. "Thread is made of cotton. Handkerchiefs may look different but the cotton in them is the same." Like us, he said. "All of us are God."

I'd read this teaching of his in Dr. Sandweiss's book. But I didn't feel it. I mustered some courage and, shaking, raised my hand. "I don't feel like God," I mumbled. Baba looked right at me and told me to see God in myself and in everyone. He told me to practice *sadhana*: spiritual rituals such as meditation, the *japamala* (rosary), and repeating God's name. I promised myself I would try.

Next, he spoke to an elderly gentleman who was losing his vision. Baba told him not to worry. Baba made several small quick circular movements with his hand and, right in front of my eyes, a silver ring materialized in his palm. I sat directly under his hand, and I was certain he'd had nothing up his sleeve. He handed the ring to the man. It bore an enamel image of Sai

Baba's head and fit the man's ring finger perfectly. Baba asked the devotee if he'd prefer to have Jesus's face. Stunned, the guy nodded "yes." Baba took back the ring, closed it in his fist, and blew on it three times. *Poof.* The ring now featured an enamel portrait of Jesus. *Holy shit!* A young Indian woman pulled from her purse a tiny pouch containing an aquamarine gemstone. She handed it to Baba and asked him to bless it. He folded his hand around the stone and blew. When he opened his hand, the stone was the size of a half-dollar and it was set in gold and hanging on a chain. I'd read about these miracles, but to witness them blew my mind. I left the interview room in a daze.

My head spinning, I decided to search for the dogs. Each day I'd skipped lunch at the canteen and headed to the bakery, where I bought a few loaves for the dogs and me. Although my bulimia had spun out of control in Italy, here in India, surrounded by starving people and animals, the thought of binging, let alone vomiting it up, felt selfish and repugnant. Instead, I decided to limit my dietary intake, not like an anorectic, but enough to reach my idealized weight of 110 pounds, which I hadn't seen since I was seventeen. Whole-wheat bread, plus a few protein-laden nuts, available from the ashram's kiosks, seemed perfect.

I'd located several dog dens on the edges of the ashram. Each time I arrived with the bread, the dogs would form a circle around me, and, like perfect ladies and gentlemen, would delicately accept the food from my hands. If they were too nervous, I'd toss it gently at their feet.

On the tenth day, my last at the ashram, I sat in the Darshan line and wrote a letter, a prayer really, straight from my heart. I prayed for help with my bulimia. I prayed for faith. I prayed I'd graduate from vet school. And although it felt like *chutzpa*, I prayed for a sign that God heard my prayer. I held out my letter as Baba passed. He took it but didn't open it. Instead, he said, "Come." He gestured toward the marble verandah where a few others waited for a private *private* interview.

I entered the interview room and sat on the floor in a semi-circle with half a dozen others. He called us one by one into an even smaller rear room. When it was my turn, he stood barely a foot or two from me. He looked up.

"Marcie, how are you?"

He knew my name! I managed a weak smile. "Good."

He knew otherwise. He told me I was anxious, worried, and nervous. All true. He said my mind was always leaping like a monkey from here to there. True again. He told me he knew my heart had just been broken. How did he know my best friend had stolen the only man I had ever loved? He told me not to worry; he would give me a good life.

We walked out together into the main room and took our seats. Then, Baba turned to me and spoke. I couldn't make out the words. Baba repeated. Still, I was confused.

"Samuel Sandweiss," someone translated, pointing to an older gentleman across the aisle.

Out of the tens of thousands of people present at the ashram on that particular day in December 1980, I was sitting in the same tiny room as Dr. Samuel Sandweiss of San Diego, the psychiatrist who'd written the book that had led me here in the first place! When the interview ended, I dashed out to find Dr. Sandweiss. I knew Baba had directed me to him for help. I told the doctor that I had bulimia and that I hadn't sought professional help for my eating disorder, because I feared analysts would ridicule my spiritual search. Under a palm tree, outside his small room in the ashram, the doctor encouraged me to seek help, and I determined on the spot that I would.

Before we boarded the bus, I ran to my dogs to say goodbye and to offer them one last meal.

Chapter 5

From Butcher to Binger

When I returned to Italy, my soul was on fire.

I made a plan. First, I promised God that I would never eat meat again. I'd been a reluctant vegetarian since I was seventeen, because I didn't want to eat the animals I loved. But in Italy, when faced with a plate of *norcina*—orecchiette pasta, ground pork, cremini mushrooms, heavy cream, white wine, and nutmeg—my willpower often failed me.

Second, I vowed to let go of fear and ramp up my exams.

Prior to India, I'd been semi-paralyzed by fear. Exams in Italian vet school were given monthly, at a go-at-your-own-pace system. No quizzes, no midterms, no homework. Just one final exam in each of the fifty-one courses, with hundreds of pages of notes to memorize for each. The information rarely came from textbooks; rather, it came from professors' lectures. So, like nearly all the other students, Italian and American, I relied on the piles of notes, *appunti*, written in Italian, scribbled by the few attendees. Since I could barely understand Italian, it could take me a whole day to translate one page.

Plus, I had to tackle the science.

To get into an American veterinary school I'd have needed two full years of college science. I hadn't taken a science course since high school. I prided myself on the fact that I managed to graduate from Boston University after transferring from Emory without a single science course. I hated science. It bored me. I'd only studied subjects that interested me and ended up with a major in philosophy and a minor in literature.

In Bologna, an exam consisted of three random questions from an entire course, asked orally, in Italian, in front of a hundred or more students. To pass, the questions needed to be answered nearly perfectly and out loud, in Italian.

Oy veh.

Knowing the material backward and forward and inside-out didn't mean one would pass. Often, passing or failing seemed to depend more on the mood of the professor than on a student's knowledge.

Prior to India, I'd sat in one *appello* (exam session) where the professor laughed and joked, and every student passed. Then he abruptly left to take a phone call and came back fuming. The rest of the class flunked. I sat that one out and took it the following month.

During another exam, a professor threw my friend John's *libretto* (report card) out the window and told him—and the class—that John should study law because he'd never be a vet.

To figure out how to address my second vow, I scrutinized the students who flew through their exams—all the Israelis and some of the Italians. I noticed that they tended to study in pairs.

I found an Italian, Cristiana. Or I should say, Cristiana found me.

The blond-haired, blue-eyed beauty approached me one day and introduced herself. For some reason she wanted to study with me. Great! An Italian study partner—she'd have all the *appunti*.

During our first study date, she told me she had only two exams left.

"How did you pass so many exams?" I said, stunned. We were both in our fifth and (supposedly) final year of vet school, and I still had thirty-eight exams to go.

She grinned. "I'm dating *Professore* Rossi." He was middle-aged and married.

I'd heard rumors about girls sleeping with their teachers for *racommendazioni,* or a passing grade.

"I can help you," she said with a sly smile. "The *professore* wanted me to speak to you. He's good friends with Professor Morro, who thinks you're very pretty. He wants to ask you out." Another married guy.

So *that's* why Cristiana had sought me out! I'd heard that Professor Morro recommended a lot of American girls, passing them no matter their knowledge of the material.

I thought of the dozens of exams I had yet to pass. I looked at Cristiana's radiant face. She had only two left. I hesitated. "Umm, *va bene* (OK)," I mumbled, scared out of my wits.

I agreed to meet the *professore,* only if Cristiana came along for the meet and greet. And only in the daytime, outside his lecture hall.

Come noon, on The Day, I pulled on a low-cut, black, clingy rayon dress and laid on the make-up. I checked myself in the full-length mirror, took a deep breath, and then wobbled my way to the bus stop in my spikey high heels.

Light-headed, with butterflies battering my stomach, I neared the pre-arranged meeting point on campus—the courtyard outside the old brick building where Morro lectured. An ebullient Cristiana and a short and swarthy Dr. Morro stood waiting.

Feeling faint and slightly nauseated, I inched forward. Morro sidled right up. *"Allora, quando noi usciamo*? (So, when are we going out?)" He smirked.

I looked down at him from my high heels and paused. Could I really sell my soul (or my body) for a passing grade?

"Mai! (Never!)" I blurted out. I tore off my heels and ran.

Back to the books.

Cristiana out of the picture, I created a rigid study schedule for myself. I rose at 3 a.m., just as I had in India. I stood next to my platform bed in clogs and sweatpants, textbook or notes perched on the bedspread. I propped a framed photo of Sai Baba on the bed next to my notes. I'd chosen that photo because Baba seemed to look straight into my eyes, like he had at the ashram—a reminder that God was with me. Each morning, before I'd start to memorize, I stared into those eyes and said a prayer. I had to memorize lists and lists. Lists of diseases, lists of etiologies, lists of drugs, lists of body parts, lists of lists. I felt as if I were memorizing the telephone directory.

To keep focused, I came up with what I hoped was a fail-proof method. First, I underlined every single word with a blue ballpoint pen. On the second go-round, I used a red ballpoint to squiggle under important words. Then I used different colored highlighters for the third, fourth, fifth, and sixth readings: blue for section titles, green for subtitles, orange for key words, and yellow for all the rest. All six times I read the information out loud so I wouldn't fall asleep. I lived on Halls menthol lozenges.

And not much else.

During my almost five years in Bologna, I continued to struggle with the bulimia that had plagued me since college at Emory University when my freshman roommate, a beautiful southern belle and homecoming queen, had shared this weight control method with me. I'd managed to keep my bulimia in check until my second exam in vet school, Anatomy I. I'd spent a year preparing for that exam. We had to identify bones, parts of bones, ligament attachments to bones, and everything to do with equine and bovine bones for the practical section of the exam. I'd actually attended one of the labs. Dozens of students had crowded around the few available bones. I couldn't see a thing. Not knowing where to turn, I left. I'd need to assemble my own skeletons, both horse and cow.

I found a couple of butchers, one regular and one specializing in horse-meat, and begged them for bones. I needed them all: femur, tibia, scapula, radius, and, in particular, I needed a horse's head. The horse butcher smiled. He disappeared in the back and returned with an entire horse's head with a metal ring through its nostrils, hanging in a bucket. "I have to cut all the meat off first," he stressed.

"Please do," I said, bile rising in my mouth.

I carried everything home, piece by piece. I boiled the body parts, one at a time, on my kitchen stove in a huge vat I'd collected from a gas station. Then I hosed down the bones in my bathtub, making sure to pick off all the flesh.

I'd held myself together until I had to pull the brain out through the eye sockets—then I puked. I suspect even non-vegetarians would've had that problem. My apartment stank for weeks, but I did learn the bones. As did the many other students who borrowed my increasingly famous collection.

That turned out to be the easy part. It took months to memorize the material. By the time I reached the end of the notes, I'd forgotten the beginning. Mentally, I broke down. It got to the point where whenever I sat in front of the mountain of papers, my mind and body balked. To defer and delay, I'd run to the refrigerator and binge. Usually on whole wheat Weight

Watchers crackers (yes, there was a Weight Watchers in Bologna) that I'd spread with butter and honey (the only temptation I'd allow in my apartment). Stopping eating meant returning to the books, so I'd continue to stuff myself. Gaining weight was not an option, so I brought up almost all that I'd swallowed.

Despite my vows, upon my return from India, I continued to struggle. My dread of exams triggered binge/purge cycles. I had managed to take and pass only one exam by the time summer break rolled around.

It was time to follow Dr. Sandweiss's advice and find a psychiatrist, to keep my second vow.

Chapter 6

Ten Weeks to Chutzpa

In June, I went home to Lido Beach in Long Island, New York. Mom (short, pale, red-haired, and flabby) and Dad (tall, handsome, and smiling) met me at arrivals at JFK International Airport. Mom, who didn't like to show her emotions, squelched a flush of delight that darted across her face. Dad planted a wet one on my cheek. I cringed.

When I passed across the threshold of our house on Regent Drive, I felt like I'd stepped back into my childhood, even though I was twenty-eight years old. Back to an overly critical mother, an angry and misanthropic father, and a twenty-six-year-old sister who hated me. The fighting started in minutes. In short order, I decided to move into my Grandma Betty's studio apartment at the Carnegie House at 100 West 57th Street in New York City. My sanctuary.

I adored Grandma Betty. From the time I was twelve, when my parents allowed me to ride the train by myself, I'd escape to her apartment. Twenty years later, nothing seemed different at the Carnegie House. My grandmother was one of the first tenants, and everyone loved her. The white-gloved doorman with the brown uniform trimmed in gold gave me a nod of recognition and bowed as he opened the door. The two concierges smiled as I walked past the front desk. They knew I was her granddaughter, and I felt special because of it.

Suitcase in hand, like thousands of times before, I rushed out of the elevator and down the carpeted hallway, with the familiar thrill of anticipation. I pressed the doorbell at 4L. Grandma's face glowed as she opened the door. She wore a simple, decades-old, red-and-white-checkered suit, carrying herself like the queen of England. With her ramrod straight back and regal bearing, she appeared a lot taller than her five-feet one-inch. Bending down to kiss her cool cheek, I entered, inhaling the comforting fragrance of her apartment.

"Come, sit down, take your shoes off, and take a load off your feet," she quipped, pointing to her six-foot-long blue-silk-covered couch. "Let me make you some tea. I baked my 'fist' cookies especially for you."

She disappeared into the kitchenette and returned a moment later with a wooden tray laden with an antique china plate filled with my favorite cookies: rich, crumbly, butter and almond obelisks that were three inches long, wearing the imprints of her fingers. After carefully setting the tray on the marble coffee table, she sat beside me. She reached down for my feet, nestled them on her lap, and began to massage them. "Tell me all about Italy," Grandma said.

And so I did, the tension draining from my body, the stress of Lido Beach and its constant fighting, and of Bologna and its exams, melting away.

Together, after dinner, we made up the couch with fresh sheets and her colorful hand-crocheted afghan blanket. Grandma went to sleep in her twin bed in the narrow alcove, and I lay on my couch/bed. Back in my safe zone, I wrapped my *japalmala* (prayer beads) around my fingers and focused on the photo of Sai Baba I'd placed on the coffee table. To the soundtrack of Grandma's snoring, I reviewed my life's direction.

I'd ended up in Italian veterinary school by default and by choice. After college, I'd decided to pursue my childhood dream and train horses. I took a job at a show jumping barn in upstate New York. They gave me a place to sleep in a loft above the stable in exchange for one riding lesson a day. I spent ten to twelve hours a day shoveling manure, which I didn't mind. (In fact, I'd never slept better in my life!) It was my coworkers—alcoholics and drug addicts—who helped me to understand that this wasn't my career path. I left a week later.

At a loss for what to do next, I did the three things in life I'd sworn I'd never do: live with my parents, commute to New York City, and work as a secretary. (My parents and grandmother had insisted I learn stenography and typing in high school, just in case.) It wasn't all bad. I discovered ballet and attended classes at the Morelli Ballet Studio in Greenwich Village after work, five days a week. Maybe I could become a dancer! I dared to share my new passion with Mom.

"You'll never be a dancer, you're too old," she said. Instead, she told me what she'd said before I went to work with the horses: "Go to vet school."

You never want me to be happy! I wanted to scream. But I didn't. Controlling and overbearing Mom always thought she was right, and she usually was.

So, at twenty-three years old, feeling that time was running out, I listened to Mom.

In short order, my mother discovered through the Jewish grapevine that lots of Americans attended Italian veterinary schools. Generally, they'd chosen Italy because of its open enrollment policy (meaning anybody, even those with bad grades, could get in.) More importantly for me, Italy didn't mandate science prerequisites—they incorporated them into their five-year program. Besides, *Italia* seemed much more exciting than science! I couldn't wait to board the plane.

Now, five years later, in my sacred space, on Grandma's couch, muffled traffic noises from Sixth Avenue seeping through the closed windows, I asked myself the dreaded question: *how on earth can I get through this?*

I'd met Americans who'd languished in Bologna for decades. Decades! Although they'd never admitted to officially dropping out, they hadn't taken exams for years. Most got by teaching English to Italians. I avoided them like the plague.

In the morning, I asked Grandma for the Yellow Pages.

A for Anorexia? B for Bulimia? I didn't know where to begin. I opened the book and by some miracle I landed upon Dr. John Adams Atchley, president of the Anorexia and Bulimia Society of New York. I called for an appointment.

A few days later, I made my way to his office on East 68th Street, enjoying the walk through my favorite part of Manhattan. Down Central Park South, past the Plaza Hotel on my right, a favorite since Grandma had regaled me as a child with stories of Eloise, the fictitious six-year-old who lived in the penthouse. I looked left toward the horse-drawn carriages lining Central Park, their nose-bagged presence bittersweet, and whispered a little prayer for their well-being. I turned north onto Fifth Avenue, past FAO Schwartz, the famous toy store. Growing up, Grandma had taken me there each Christmas to see their holiday display. I'd stand in awe, enthralled by the almost life-sized stuffed animals: giraffes, lions, bears, and horses.

I peeked into the window of my favorite hotel, the Sherry Netherland, with its nineteenth century charm. It transported me to the days of Edith Wharton and the Gilded Age, around when Grandma was born. I continued north on Fifth Avenue to 68th Street and down the stairs to Dr. Atchley's office in an elegant Upper East Side brownstone.

I rang the bell. Dr. Atchley himself welcomed me in. Sixty-ish, he was tall, lanky, and handsome in a gray-haired Waspy way, a sort of Jimmy Stewart look-alike. He was the antithesis of my preconception of a psychiatrist.

We took our seats in two leather armchairs across from each other.

I had to ask. "Are you related to *the* John Adams?"

"Yeah, I'm great-great-great-great grand something. That and a dime will get me a phone call."

What a sweetheart. I'd hit the jackpot.

I set up weekly appointments for the ten weeks I'd be in town, every Wednesday at 11 a.m. He encouraged me to join his weekly anorexia/bulimia group therapy sessions as well. "You will get more out of the group than individual therapy with me," he insisted. "To tell you the truth, I feel like an eavesdropper. It's a privilege the women allow me in. I learn more from them than the other way around."

Never a group person, my instinct was to resist. But he persisted.

What an amazing group of women! When I mentioned my passion for ballet, one of the women, a director in the new medium called "cable TV," told me she'd introduce me to her godmother, Agnes DeMille. Another, despite her frightening skeletal appearance, was particularly astute—she'd uncover any ploy in our narratives. Turns out she wrote an advice column for the hottest magazine for teens at the time.

We were all perfectionists saddled with low self-esteem and terror of failure. Driven to be good, we'd never turn to drink or drugs. Instead, we turned to food. Perfectionists that we were, we'd never allow ourselves to be fat. In fact, we had to have what we thought was the perfect body. We either starved ourselves (anorexia) or binged and purged (bulimia).

Even though I knew it was cuckoo, I envied the anorexics' self-control. I'd managed to fast for a couple of days during college, but I lacked the willpower of anorectics. Unable to go for prolonged periods without food, I'd binge and purge, just like another member of our group, a gorgeous runway model. She'd finally met the man of her dreams on a first date. Midway through their meal at a posh restaurant, she excused herself to go to the restroom where she vomited up all she'd eaten. When the toilet overflowed and she stood ankle-deep in her undigested meal, on the most important date of her life, she realized she needed help. We identified and had a good laugh.

Not wanting this wonderful group of women to go to waste, I suggested we meet one evening for dinner. Everyone looked stunned, but they agreed.

I was the only one to see the humor, both during the meal and in the dedicated post-dinner group therapy session. Seems everyone had silently tallied how many nuts and pretzels they ate or didn't eat while we waited with our drinks, and how many calories we consumed as we picked at our meals.

These women had been in therapy for years. I had no time to waste. I had a ten-week vacation in which to heal and thirty-eight exams to pass when I returned to Bologna.

I learned a lot from these eleven attractive, articulate, over-achieving women. Over the weeks, I discovered the keys to overcoming my eating disorder: taking risks and risking failure. In other words, *chutzpa*.

I realized that was the second thing about the students in Italy who graduated on time. They didn't feel they had to know everything. They figured that since the *professore* asked only three questions, they'd study only three things. Eventually, they reasoned, the professor would get so sick of looking at their faces, he'd pass them. Those students had *chutzpa*.

By the time I took Alitalia back to Bologna, I was ready to find myself some.

Chapter 7

Partners, Pallini, and Prosciutto

Back in Bologna, I decided to prepare for the physics exam. Many Italian students considered this one of the easier tests. But I remembered physics from high school, when physics was for boys with slide rules and protractors. The geniuses.

I devised a plan unheard of in Italy: I found myself a private tutor, an Italian physics grad student who looked like he'd probably carried around slide rules and protractors in high school. I met with him twice weekly, and after just one month of preparation, I sailed through the test.

The next exam I'd heard was relatively easy was "autopsy." Professor Morro's course! I prayed he wouldn't take his revenge and fail me. I studied three short weeks, said a heartfelt prayer, and tip-toed into his classroom. He asked me three fair questions, which I answered (in Italian, as always). He passed me, probably because he never wanted to see me again.

I didn't want to put off physiology any longer, the *big* one, bigger than anatomy even. This particular professor was notorious for failing students, so I knew that preparing for this exam would test my bulimia as well.

I gathered the relevant *appunti* and books. I rose at 3 a.m. and memorized until 7 a.m., when the neighborhood coffee bar opened. Visions of a fresh baked croissant (or two) and a double cappuccino carried me through the early morning hours. After breakfast, I jogged around the block four times, one kilometer per lap, deliberately passing the upscale riding stable I'd discovered. I repeated the same mantra lap after lap. *One day I'll be a vet who can afford a horse.* Sometimes I'd take my roommate's German

Shepherd, Beppe, along. People had advised me not to take on Paola as a roommate, because of her dog. But Beppe was the best part of Paola. Smart as a whip, he never needed a leash when we jogged together. He always turned his head both ways to check the traffic before crossing the street. (However, I *had* disagreed with Paola on what to feed Beppe. I had screamed and nearly fainted the first time I lifted the lid of the pot boiling on the stove and eight chicken heads stared up at me. That and white rice, Paola insisted, was the perfect dog food.)

After jogging, I returned to the books. I *had* to know this material perfectly. The professor terrified me. What if I failed?

The ten therapy sessions seemed to keep my bulimia in check. Instead, I now obsessed about other things. *Did I lock the door?* I'd go back and check it and check it. *Did I turn off the gas stove properly?* I would turn and turn and turn the knob. Maybe this was hereditary. My father checked doorknobs constantly. He once turned the front doorknob so hard it fell off in his hands. We all made fun of him.

Now I was doing the same thing. I tried offsetting this obsessive-compulsive behavior by invoking the Divine. I'd use a holy number while I counted. I'd been told in India that 108 was the holiest number. I knew that I couldn't turn a knob 108 times due to time constraints, so I settled on second best—nine—another holy number, apparently. One. Two. Three. Four. Five. Six. Seven. Eight. Nine. I counted and invoked the Divine as I checked the stove (held off the knob and counted to nine), turned the front door handle (and counted to nine), touched the garage door (and counted to nine), and so on.

My OCD didn't stop at home. If I saw a coat schlumping unevenly over someone's chair while out to dinner with friends, I had to straighten it out. I'd pretend to need the ladies room and rearrange the coat on my way past the chair of the unknown and unknowing guest.

As time went on, my *pallini* (literally "little balls" or obsessive thoughts) multiplied exponentially. Anything could trigger this: a crack on the wall, a tear in my stockings, a bad haircut. I'd obsess for hours, days.

I figured out a solution. Since it was impossible to fixate on two things at the same time, when I started to obsess on one thing, I'd think of a second thing that bothered me and the two thoughts would cancel each other out.

I knew I was nuts, but I least I didn't vomit.

I memorized *everything* for the physiology exam. The only topic I couldn't find *appunti* for was the EKG. I asked everyone I knew. "He never asks it," they told me. "Never." I worried and obsessed, but after eleven months of studying, I knew the rest of the material backward and forward, inside and out.

"*Signorina* Fallek." On the day of the exam, the professor called me up for my three questions. I stood in front of the lecture hall and my classmates, ready and confident. Question one: blah blah. Perfect answer! Question Two: blah blah blah. Perfect answer again! Question Three: blah blah blah blah. Perfect answer yet again! Smiling and euphoric, I waited for my perfect grade of *Trenta* (thirty).

The man smiled as he added an unheard of fourth question. "*Signorina*, tell me all about the EKG."

I staggered out of the room, dizzy from the first academic failure of my life.

Somehow, I made it to the nearest *pasticceria*. "*Mi dai un cappuccino doppio e un tiramisù per favore?*" I said, requesting from the *barista* a double cappuccino and a tiramisu. I waited at the counter while the *barista* steamed the milk extra hot and plated my consolation prize. I spotted a lone table by the window. Sipping my coffee, I sought some spiritual solace.

I'd failed. But I didn't die. In fact, I didn't seem any worse for it. Like every other exam, the physiology test would be given the next month, and each month after that. I'd find some EKG notes and try again next month.

Instead of mounting the gerbil wheel of self-punishment, this time I searched for something positive. I discovered a ballet class for adults, taught by Carla, an ex-ballerina from the internationally known *La Scala*. Every Saturday morning and three nights a week, I took an hour-long bus ride to the studio. The adrenaline rush lasted through the following day.

In the meantime, I discovered obscure information about EKGs hidden in various textbooks. When I showed up for my second attempt at physiology with the same professor a month later, the first question he asked was about the EKG. I passed.

My Israeli friends had pointed out years before that if I'd divided my perfect *trentas* (thirties) by eighteen (the minimum passing score), I would have finished more exams. They'd tried to convince me that once I was a vet, no one would care what grade I'd received in school. It took a literal failure for me to face my fear of failing, and with it, my compulsion to memorize every single thing for every single test. What a waste of time!

Oh well, lesson learned. Only thirty-five more exams to go. I turned to my Israeli friend, Gy, a pre-med student, for suggestions on how to move forward. Like most Israelis, she had an opinion.

"Why don't you study with me in *Centro*, at the *Archiginassio* (public library)? I'd love the company."

That was a great idea, as it would get me out of my apartment. We couldn't be study partners, because Gy was pre-med, but this was the next best thing. Her optimism and *joie de vivre* always lifted my spirits.

We met at Piazza Maggiore, the main square of Bologna, the very next day. Gy gave me a bear hug and slid her arm through mine, steering me toward the shops lining the piazza.

"Look at these beautiful *negozi*," she said. (She was right: Italians could make a window full of socks look good.) "Stop worrying so much. Life is full of worries. When you graduate, and you will, you'll have other problems. You're in Italy. Look up. Look at the buildings. You always stare at the ground. Look up and be happy!"

Baba had said the same thing.

"Be happy."

Gy led me up worn medieval stone steps into the *Archiginassio*, and into another world. Built in the sixteenth century, the library had soaring ceilings with ancient-looking leather books lining hundreds of shelves. Long wooden-plank tables filled the cavernous space. An occasional green-shaded lamp with a twenty-watt bulb punctuated the gloom. Saving electricity at the expense of eyesight. So Italian. Gy found us two seats together on one of the attached benches, thankfully, near a lamp.

I opened my *appunti* and stared down at my notes. An uncontrollable urge for something chocolate seized me. I couldn't concentrate. *Infectious diseases of chickens*: *Avian flu, avian tuberculosis, chlamydiosis* . . . Sacher torte or cannoli? Or maybe just an Italian hot chocolate, like melted dark-chocolate pudding, the kind you had to eat with a spoon.

I glanced at Gy and then bolted out the door and down the stairs to Zanarini's, the best *pasticerria* in Bologna. I'd decided on the Sacher torte, a dense rich chocolate cake coated with dark chocolate icing, hold the whipped cream. I inhaled the *torta*, washed it down with a latte, and ran back to my post. Gy looked up. I shrugged and turned back to my notes.

Avian encephalomyelitis, coccidiosis, cryptosporidiosis . . . Damn, the librarians wouldn't shut up. They chattered on as if they were in their own home. Plus, the hall echoed as bad as the special tunnel in Piazza Maggiore that drew droves of tourists. I needed absolute quiet to concentrate. Even a ticking clock drove me crazy.

I strode to the counter, fuming, but in my most polite tone, asked, "Could you please keep your voices down? I am trying to study."

They glared at me like I was some kind of alien and returned to their conversation.

Basta! Enough! Despite Gy's comforting presence, no way could I study there.

The next day, I had another idea. Traffic noise calmed me. Like white noise. Like my sound machine. I bundled up, grabbed my book, and headed for *Centro*. Miles of porticos covered the Bolognese streets, almost forty kilometers of them to be exact. Built in the Middle Ages to support the extra living space of the upper floors of homes, porticos had the added benefit of protecting man and beast and me from the elements: rain, snow, wind, and sun. Open book in hand, I pounded the pavement, crossing streets, from portico to portico, dodging the rain.

I memorized out loud the causes of diarrhea in chickens. No one seemed to notice me talking to myself or maybe I didn't notice because I concentrated so well. Either way, it worked. I was able to memorize.

I'd wind my way through the cobble-stoned streets, staring down at my book. I'd lift my eyes every so often to admire a particularly attractive *vetrina*. If I spotted one of Bologna's many medieval churches, I'd step into the dimly lit gothic space to light a candle and say a prayer—"Please God, help me pass my exam"—before continuing on my way.

With all these porticos, I couldn't get bored. I walked six hours a day. Movement focused me almost as well as my mother's weight-shedding amphetamines had. All of Bologna's fabulous coffee bars and *pasticcerias* lay at my feet, so there was no mad dash down library stairs for caffeine or chocolate. No guilt either. If I stopped for a treat, I'd burn off the calories. I killed two birds with one stone.

This gave me another idea. If walking worked, perhaps train rides would also.

Through ballet, I'd met a group of Italian women who'd invited me to join them on their expeditions to ballet performances around Italy. Although tempted, I'd turned them down, because I'd feel guilty wasting time not studying. I rethought the situation. These girls always took the train. Motion calmed my nerves, and the chugging engines made a white noise. On the train, I couldn't make a pit stop at a bakery or coffee bar, so I decided to join them. While these women talked among themselves and dreamed of ballet and *danseurs*, I studied. Obstetrics, pharmacology, propaedeutics, teratology . . . And while they watched Bejart perform in *Venezia*, the Paris Opera dance in *Reggio Emilia*, and Nureyev perform at La Scala in *Milano*, I dozed.

I made some headway.

But not enough. I was now two years *fuori corso*, two years beyond the five-year program, with twenty exams completed and thirty-one to go.

I turned to Gy again. "Get a study partner, this time, a fat, ugly one," said Gy, who was overweight and stunning.

Letizia fit the bill. She was mousy with stringy brown hair, wore thick glasses —and had the latest *appunti*. We planned on studying toxicology together at her apartment. She'd prepare lunch. On the first day, we settled down to study at her kitchen table. Then I heard it.

"What's that?" I said.

"What's what?"

"That chirping."

"Does it bother you?"

"Yes!"

Letizia rolled her eyes. "Look outside."

I got up and stuck my head out the window. A pair of blue parakeets chirped merrily from a cage hung outside her neighbors' window. "They're making a racket," I said. "I can't focus. Can you please call those people and tell them to take the birds inside?"

"Marcie, relax. Don't let two little *uccellini* bother you. Focus on your work."

Truth be told, I wished I had a slingshot… Some vet I'd make!

When lunchtime rolled around, Letizia busied herself at the stove.

"I prepared you a Tuscan specialty."

Great, I was starving!

Smiling, she set down a plate of steaming pasta in front of me. My eyes narrowed. "What are those little brown *pezzi* in the penne?"

"Prosciutto."

"I told you, I don't eat meat."

"That's not meat; it's prosciutto."

For reasons I couldn't understand, Italians didn't consider prosciutto meat. I think they considered it a condiment, like *sale* and pepper. But it *was* meat. I even knew how to cure and dry it, thanks to *Tecnica Conserviera* and *Ispezione e controllo delle derrate alimentare di origine animale* (Conservation and Inspection of Food of Animal Origin*),* which taught us how to make prosciutto. We learned not only how to can dead animals, but also how to make the cans. It had never occurred to me that we'd study animals as part of the food chain! We even took a field trip to the slaughterhouse for *Lavori Pratici nei Macelli* (Practical Work in Slaughterhouses), as veterinarians had to certify that a slaughterhouse was sanitary, that the animals were healthy before slaughter, and that when they ended up on our dinner table, they were free of germs and contaminants.

In fact, the only time I'd seen live animals in Italian vet school was at the slaughterhouse. And they didn't last long there. Just until the retractable, reusable bullet entered the cow's head. Or the pig's throat was slit as the conveyer belt grabbed its rear leg. This wasn't the kind of veterinary work I wanted any part of. My goal was to help heal these creatures. At Letizia's table, I sent a silent prayer of thanks to those mangy Indian dogs, which had reminded me why I'd started this quest. It sure wasn't to learn to make sausages and salami.

Despite the birds and prosciutto, Letizia and I made a great team. We passed three exams together.

Chapter 8

The Doctor Makes a Deal

I had to pee all the time. I'd had an overactive bladder long before vet school. A minor surgical procedure had addressed it in the past, but the urologist at the time had warned me that the trouble would return. I hadn't seen a doctor yet in Italy, but I couldn't put it off any longer.

I headed over to San Orsola Hospital. The receptionist ushered me into an enormous exam room, where I waited and fretted for almost an hour, concerned about losing study time.

A tall, dark, and handsome man with bushy eyebrows entered. He wore a white lab coat with a stethoscope curled around his neck. He smiled, extended his hand, and introduced himself: Dr. Berman, head of the Urology Department. Israeli, I could tell by his accent. Gorgeous. My anxiety vanished.

After I explained my condition, he gestured toward an exam chair, the one with the stirrups. No changing room. No disposable paper gown. Not even a sheet. I had to remove my jeans and underwear right there, alone with him, while he watched. Then I took a seat in the saddle.

"How do you like living in Italy?" he asked, clearly delighted to speak with a fellow foreigner.

We discussed living as expats in Italy as I dissociated myself from the lower half of my body and he examined my vagina.

Just then a group of medical students, young men around my age, entered. They were apparently on a clinical rotation for OBGYN. The five guys lined up behind Dr. B, who interrupted his exam and introduced them to me one by one. Was he kidding? I forced myself to answer their oddly animated questions about life in New York, while suppressing the sensation that I was the subject of a photo shoot for *Playboy Magazine*.

When the students finally left, Dr. B straightened up and walked over to a desk. Avoiding his eyes, I dismounted the table, pulled on my underpants and jeans and sat on the chair across from him. He looked up from his notes and smiled. I managed a frozen half-smile.

We set a date for surgery, which later went smoothly.

At our post-surgical appointment, Dr. B asked if I could help him translate a few paragraphs from Italian to English for a book he was writing.

"Of course," I murmured.

We met at a cafe on campus the next week to review his chapter.

He looked at me intently. "Thanks so much for your help. What can I do to repay the favor?"

Had I imagined it, or had his hand lingered over mine as he handed over the document?

"*Niente* (nothing)," I said, hoping he would ask me out for a date.

"Don't you have any difficult exams you need help with?"

I looked at him, confused, until clarity dawned. "Well there *are* a few." Of my twenty-nine remaining exams, six were given by notoriously unpredictable professors.

"Let me know when you decide to take them, and I'll take care of the rest," the doctor said.

A few days prior to each of the six exams, I called Dr. B and told him both the professor and the date of the exam. I had no idea what would transpire between them, and I studied diligently as usual.

During each of those exams, the professors asked me three questions in a perfectly professional manner, and I answered them in kind. That I passed each one was the only peculiarity.

Finally, I had graduation in my sights! Then, three months before I hoped to graduate, my friend Laurie asked how my thesis was coming along.

"What thesis?"

"You need to present a paper in Italian at graduation. That *is* the graduation. A panel of professors will ask you questions about your thesis."

How did I not know this? I'd managed to pass more than twenty exams in one year and was counting the days to graduation. "Did you write yours yet?" I said.

"Are you kidding?" she scoffed. "Angela's doing it."

"Who?"

"Angela! She's an Italian medical student who supports herself by writing theses for Americans."

A medical mercenary. Brilliant!

Two months later, on May 27, 1986, I sat for my last exam: *Idrobiologia e Piscicoltura*, in other words, "fish." I memorized dozens and dozens of species of fish. Mostly, I learned how to differentiate between species: eye placement, fins, color, shape of head, tail, mouth, and anything else needed to tell one fish from another.

I entered the *aula* and took my seat across the desk from the *professore*, an elderly bald man with kind eyes, who looked bemused.

"*Perche sei cosi nervosa?* (Why are you so nervous?)," he asked.

"This is my last exam!" I blurted out.

"*Non preoccuparla* (don't worry), *Signorina Americana*." Still smiling, he asked, "How do you prepare shrimp in your country?"

I stared at him. This was the exam question?

He elaborated. "When you go out to dinner, do you ever order shrimp?"

"Yes," I lied. I didn't eat any meat, fish included.

"What is your favorite dish?"

"*Shrimp Scampi!*" I exclaimed, triumphant.

I passed.

I had said to myself dozens of times during my decade in Bologna that if I ever managed to graduate from Italian veterinary school, it was purely God's grace.

During my tenth and final year, I had sat for and passed twenty-six exams. The previous twenty-five exams had taken nine years.

On graduation day, I entered the grand *aula* dressed in my brand new white and black Christian Dior silk polka dot dress that I'd snapped up on sale. Shaking, I handed a beautifully bound copy of "Mammary Tumors in

Dogs" to each of the five professors seated at the semi-circular table, then took my seat across from them.

I began to read my thesis. When I looked up halfway through my presentation, three of the five appeared to be dozing off. Only the woman with a crewcut and my advisor, a handsome, bearded man, seemed to be paying attention. The latter winked at me and gave an encouraging smile. When I finished, the other three shook themselves awake long enough to ask me a few perfunctory questions. Ten minutes later, it was over. I shook their hands, smiling broadly.

Now I was officially a veterinarian, with a degree from *l'Università di Bologna Scuola di Medicina Veterinaria*. Hallelujah!

After graduation, Dr. Berman explained the deal he'd struck with those six professors. If I knew the material, I would pass. If I didn't, I'd fail.

That had been my prayer all along.

(Ten years later, I received notice that my diploma was ready for retrieval at the registrar's office. Huge and tasteful and in color. It was beautiful, but ten years late. So Italian.)

Chapter 9

An Alternate Reality

I boarded an Alitalia flight from Milan to New York, flush with victory. I couldn't wait to return to the United States, to a world that functioned logically and efficiently. A world filled with air-conditioning and public restrooms with actual toilets versus holes in the floor.

I spotted my parents just outside the red velvet security rope in arrivals at JFK airport and rushed over. After we said our hellos, Mom said, "So what took you so long?"

My jaw tightened. "What is that supposed to mean?"

"It means it took you ten years to finish a five-year program!"

I bit my lip and kept silent. I didn't expect a party, but a "congratulations" would have been nice.

I trailed my parents to baggage claim, where, to my horror, I discovered that my six pieces of luggage and old camp trunk had not arrived.

"Lost," somebody told us.

My head buzzed. "What the hell . . ."

"We'll deal with that later," Mom cut in. "I'm tired, I want to go home."

I rolled my eyes as soon as she turned away, hoping she didn't notice.

Shoulders sagging, I fell into a slouch sure to trigger Mom's ire. I felt like a twelve-year-old. I walked at least ten paces behind my parents as we made our way to short-term parking. Mom took the wheel of our powder blue Oldsmobile, and I crawled into the back. Before starting the car, she turned to me. "So, after ten years, don't you have anything to say to us?"

"Not really." I sighed. Nothing that I'd accomplished ever seemed enough for Mommy. In high school my A's made little impact. But if she sniffed out a B+ or, God forbid, a B, she'd say, "So? What happened?" I didn't stand up straight enough. Eyebrow pencil belonged on my eyebrows, not on my lower lids. No one wears white lipstick. She had been especially angry that I didn't date during high school. She refused to believe that at fifteen no one had asked me out. She accused me of turning down all the boys just to spite her. She would never have believed that I suffered through my junior prom with a nerdy boy with pimples just to please her.

The silence of the thirty-minute drive home was broken only by Dad's screaming whenever Mom made a wrong turn.

God give me strength. Over the past ten years, rolling green farmland dotted with gray stone or red brick farmhouses in Reggio Emilia had welcomed me back to Bologna. Each time my train from Milan rounded the bend toward *Terminale Centrale*, I'd catch a glimpse of the medieval church *Chiesa San Luca*, the iconic symbol of Bologna, from my upholstered compartment. I'd feel like I was in a scene straight out of *North by Northwest*, but Italian style.

Here, though, as my parents argued, I looked out at the ugly strip malls, fast food restaurants, and gas stations that lined Rockaway Boulevard. Sirens screamed. Cars honked. I felt like I'd entered a different universe, the appalling reality that I'd forgotten. The odor of hot asphalt wafted through the open window. I felt nauseous and closed my eyes. Somehow, the street smells of India seemed more appealing.

We parked in the driveway of our colonial home, where my thirty-one-year-old sister Debra still lived. Despite a law degree and several Masters' degrees, my sister never seemed to work. Mostly she slept, watched TV, and ranted. I ran to the door and rang the bell.

"Well, look who's finally home," Debra said. She turned on her heel and stomped back to her room, with its two TV sets stacked on top of each other on the gold metal rack so she could watch two shows at the same time without getting up to change the channel.

Though she may not have believed me, I felt bad for her. Corticosteroid treatment for a childhood illness had initiated a weight problem and now she bordered on obese. She'd stopped eating with us long ago—one too many fights about her portion sizes. Her freckled face wore a perpetual scowl. I'd brought up her weight only once, when my parents criticized her meal selection at a Chinese restaurant. She turned to me, her face filled with hate. "You have an eating disorder also!"

I'd said, "At least mine works."

When Debra retreated to her room, I cornered Mom in the kitchen. "What's up with Debra? She seems worse than usual."

"Sit down," she whispered, "I'll tell you."

I felt butterflies, as Mom never confided in me.

"We had a family therapy session," Mom said.

I couldn't believe it. For years, everyone had blamed me for the fighting. But during my ten years away, apparently the fights continued.

"As soon as the session started, your father told the psychiatrist that he didn't love Debra as much as he loved you, because she wasn't thin and feminine like you," she said.

"Debra and I stormed out, furious with your father. We didn't speak to him for weeks. She probably blames you. Try to be nice to her—it's not her fault." Tears welled up in Mom's eyes.

What an awful thing to hear. I turned away, speechless. I reminded myself of Baba's words to love all and determined to try my best.

Chapter 10

Wait, More Tests?

Before I could work in the United States as a vet, I'd have to pass the American boards. I had no idea what that entailed, only that I'd need to learn the entire American Veterinary School curriculum: four years of material, much of it different from what I'd learned in Italy. I graduated with lots of theoretical knowledge, but no practical experience. I'd never performed any surgery, drawn blood, or inserted an IV catheter. In fact, I'd barely seen a live animal at vet school, except for at that slaughterhouse.

At the only small-animal lab class offered in Bologna, I'd stood behind a crowd of hundreds of students as the professor demonstrated a cat castration. My positioning turned out to be a blessing. I couldn't witness, only hear, the shriek, as the doctor castrated the cat the same way they castrated piglets: upside down in a boot, without anesthesia.

I wondered how other Bologna grads had succeeded in the States. Then I remembered Dominic, originally from New Jersey, who'd graduated from Bologna a year before me. I found his number in my address book.

"Call Joe," he told me. "He's taken the American Boards twice. He has lots of notes."

I called Joe the same day. "There's so much shit you have to know. I have a ton of material you can photocopy. Why don't you come to my apartment? I'll give you the lowdown," he offered.

I scribbled down directions to his apartment and headed to Floral Park, Queens.

A buzzer rang me in. I climbed the stairs to the second-floor flat Joe shared with his girlfriend. A short, stocky, Italian man wearing an orange T-shirt, with the words "New York City Department of Sanitation" emblazoned on it (How cool—I wanted one!), opened the door. A long-haired tiger cat stayed by his side, just like a dog would.

"Hi! Nice to meet you," he said in a strong Queens accent.

I followed Joe to the kitchen where he pulled a rickety wooden chair into the middle of the room—holding it out for me like I was royalty. He told me to wait and disappeared into a back room. I reached down to pet the cat who, purring loudly, rubbed against my legs.

Joe returned a few minutes later, carrying stacks of paper.

"See these? They're gold. Old board exams from the past five years. A guy I worked with at the racetrack gave them to me."

"But they don't give the same test every year. How is this going to help?"

"They'll give you a good idea of *how* they ask the questions. You know the material already."

I do?

"Let's go over exactly what tests you need to take."

"I want to take the California boards," I told him. Whatever my future held, I knew it wouldn't be on Long Island or New York. I'd left the States in the seventies, close enough to the sixties, that California still held me in its spell. Both LA and San Francisco had the added appeal of being three thousand miles away from my family.

"You missed the deadline. The Educational Commission for Foreign Veterinary Graduates rules just changed. You can only take the boards for New York, Connecticut, and Florida."

My jaw dropped. "You're kidding? There's no way for me to work in California?"

"There *is* a way. It ain't easy. You gotta do the fourth year of the University of Oklahoma's vet school. After that you take a three-day, three-thousand-dollar exam that no one from Italy has ever passed. But who knows? You can be the first!"

I didn't know whether to laugh or cry.

"Don't be upset," he said. "These are good states to practice in."

My life-plan had just been turned upside down. I didn't want to live in any of those states.

"Back to the boards," he continued. "First of all, you need to pass the National Board exam, valid for the three states. It's a three-hundred-question, multiple-choice test. Easy. Connecticut requires a written Clinical Competency test. It's a fun test."

I'd never found any test fun. Now I was in a bad mood.

Joe said, "The New York State exam, on the other hand, is a bitch. It's a combination oral and practical. You get three attempts to pass it. I failed twice already," he said with a grimace. "Florida's exam is the easiest—it's a take-home, open-book test on the rules and laws of veterinary medicine in Florida—so most foreign grads end up there."

All things considered, Joe said I should focus on the New York boards, a hands-on practical given over two days at Cornell. There were six stations, he told me: horses, cows, goats, sheep, pigs, chicken, and exotics. "They make you prove you know how to handle the animals," he said.

At the equine station, for example, the examiner could ask me to lift and inspect a hoof. All I knew about picking up horses' feet was that they could kick you and you could die.

Joe continued, "At the bovine section, they could ask you to hook the udder to a milking machine and turn it on." In Italy, the only time I'd seen a cow up close was at the slaughterhouse, and they sure didn't milk them there. "Or you might have to perform a mastitis test or identify farm utensils like emasculators."

I'd never heard of either, but I did remember that Italian vets used rubber bands to castrate farm animals. Joe told me he'd been asked to point to the instrument used to dehorn a cow. After ten years of vet school, I didn't even know that cows had horns. My eyes glazed over, and the Eustachian tube in my right ear closed up and buzzed.

"Don't worry," Joe said. "This is the easy stuff."

"It is?"

"Yeah, you know all the hard stuff."

"I do?"

"You just need to think like a farmer."

Oh boy. I'd never stepped foot on a farm.

"You just need to reorganize the stuff in your mind to view it from the perspective of an actual situation. Say the farmer has a herd of itchy sheep. The examiner will ask you what could cause the itching."

In Italy, my memorized lists were of diseases, not of causes of itching.

"Buy books for veterinary technicians," Joe suggested. "Those books explain what you need to know. They also have diagrams."

Joe told me that the University of Pennsylvania vet school offered a weekend crash course a month before the New York boards. Cornell and the University of Pennsylvania vet schools competed as to which was the most prestigious, he said. "Cornell intentionally teaches its students slightly different methods from UPenn so that the UPenn students can't pass New York's exam. In retaliation, UPenn set up this course to help their students pass. We can piggyback with the UPenn students. I went last year. It was fantastic!"

Though not enough to pass the test, apparently.

Joe invited me to join him and his friend Chuck for the weekend course.

"I'm nowhere near ready!" I said.

"Don't worry. You'll learn everything there that you need to know."

Learn everything in two days? Was he kidding?

Three hours later, clutching the precious stash of tests, I thanked Joe profusely.

Chapter 11

Cows Kick Sideways

On the bright side, this time I had only four-years-worth of material to learn. And it was in English.

I tried studying at home, but my habit of talking out loud while I studied disturbed my sister. Even whispering caused an outburst.

Mom invited me to accompany her to work, where I could study in a partitioned area in the back of her third-grade gifted classroom while she taught. Despite some misgivings, I agreed to give it a try.

In her classroom, outside of the family circus, Mom was a different person. Instead of defending herself from unrelenting demands and criticism from my father and sister, she basked in the respect and admiration of her students. She helped them blossom.

My mother had once dreamed of being a lawyer, like her friend Sandy. (Mom had received an unheard-of perfect score on the LSATs.) And Mom had graduated at age nineteen from New York University with a major in architecture and a minor in labor arbitration. But no one would hire a woman architect in the 1950s, and my father said he'd divorce her if she got a law degree. So, Mom did what many women in the fifties did—she got a teaching degree. And she'd made the most of it. She'd won the New York State Teacher of the Year award and became the president of her teachers union, negotiating the highest salary in the state. Mom was happy at work, and happy people are kind. In the classroom, I loved her!

Studying there worked out perfectly for me. The hubbub from the class blurred into white noise, which helped me focus. Her mini fridge, containing only diet soda and a handful of carrot and celery sticks, didn't tempt me. I could look forward to a slice of pizza with Mom for lunch. And without a car, I was captive. My workday had a beginning and an end: I started at eight with the third graders and finished with the bell, at three.

Thanks to Joe, I had hundreds and hundreds of pages of multiple-choice questions from previous exams, along with the four or five possible answers. I decided to study not only the questions, but also each answer, so I'd cover more ground. I focused on one answer at a time, studying everything I could find on that subject. I figured I could eliminate two of the four answers by logic alone. This beat the Italian, oral, three-question final exam any time.

I worried more about the practical. I'd gotten no hands-on experience in vet school, my horse's skeleton in the tub notwithstanding. Prior to Bologna, I'd volunteered for a month at our family vet's practice, where the vets had encouraged me to observe them perform surgery. But after spending a sickening (and boring) hour watching them remove a dog's anal glands, I chose to stay in the bathing area, where I washed the filthy dogs before discharging them from boarding. That experience broke my heart. I learned that we pet owners had been lied to—the dogs were never walked. Instead, they lay in the dark in their excrement for hours and sometimes days. I avoided the vets and hung out with the techs, who seemed to love animals as much as I did. When I left for vet school, the owners, one of whom was on the New York State Veterinary testing board, had told me to keep in touch. The guy had told me he could be crucial in helping me pass. But I wanted nothing more to do with him or his partner ever again. Their practice seemed heartless. It was a miracle that my stint at that hospital didn't turn me off from veterinary medicine entirely.

As far as the practical, Joe said, I'd need to focus first on cows, which were a big deal on the New York exam, apparently. I'd bottle-fed calves while volunteering at a kibbutz in Israel, but I'd never stuck my arm up a cow's rectum, which according to the notes, was how you figured out the stage of an ovary and whether it was ripe for artificial insemination.

Thank God for Joe. He had a solution for everything. He told me about a cow farmer in Herkimer, New York, who'd helped many Italian grads learn the ropes. I called the farmer, set a date, and made a reservation at a roadside motel near Herkimer for a week.

I couldn't wait to pack my bag and leave Lido Beach. Besides the opportunity to escape from my family, I loved an adventure. When the day arrived, I loaded the trunk with my blankets, pillows, and sleeping gear and climbed behind the wheel of my father's Buick. I stuck *The Best of the Beach Boys* into the cassette player, turned it on full blast, cranked down the windows, and took off. My body swayed and my foot tapped as the ocean-scented warm air and good vibrations swept me back to 1970: I was seventeen once again, the summer between high school and college, with no responsibilities and no tests.

Six hours later I checked into the motel and dropped my bag on the bed. I pulled on the new blue-jean overalls I'd bought at the Army/Navy store, traded my Keds for new green rubber boots, and hurried over to the farm.

A weedy, middle-aged man with a beard and a friendly smile waited for me inside the barn, as promised. My Wellingtons made deep sucking noises as I picked my way carefully through the mud and manure. I nearly passed out from the stench. A row of black and white spotted cows stood placidly in their stalls, noses toward the wall, rear ends facing out. The farmer leaned casually against a flank of one of them, a pail by his feet.

I moved toward the front of the Holstein to pet her. She turned her bony head toward me with curiosity.

"Have you spent much time around cows?" the farmer asked.

I looked deep into the gentle brown eyes of the Holstein and shook my head no.

I followed the farmer to the rear of the cow as he explained some basics. Farmer Jones took a shoulder-length, clear plastic glove from a pile and pulled it on. He pushed the tail to the left and schmeared the cow's rear end with some kind of lubricant. With a gentle twisting motion, he pushed his arm in as far as he could. "Easy," he said. He withdrew his arm and handed me a new glove.

Though I hardly considered myself a Jewish princess, I felt like Eva Gabor in the old TV show *Green Acres*. I had to stifle my gag reflex as I inserted my right arm into the cow's *tuches*. The farmer walked me through the process, step by step, explaining how to push gently past the pelvic rim and feel for the ovaries.

For one week I practiced. I learned about milking. I learned about hay. I learned some basic diseases. Mostly I learned about rectums (and ovaries).

The most important thing he taught me was that cows kick sideways; not all the ladies enjoyed my arm up their butts.

Despite my new-found appreciation for the sweet disposition of cows (the non-kickers, anyway), if I'd had any doubts that bovine medicine was not my calling, that week in Herkimer dispelled them. The stink of cow manure followed me back to Motel Six every evening, clinging to me despite numerous showers.

Back at Lido Beach, I moved on to dogs and cats. I figured the best way to learn about small animals was to find a job in a small-animal hospital. Despite being armed with the title "Doctor of Veterinary Medicine" earned in Bologna, I felt woefully inadequate. I lacked the most basic skills of even a veterinary technician. I hoped Italian-trained vets would understand.

I'd heard of a practice in Queens, owned by an Italian-trained couple, and went to Mom for advice.

"Why do you want to work for vets that had the same training as you? Sure, you can ask stupid questions, but you'll get stupid answers. Find a job with American-trained vets," she answered with her usual candor and common sense.

She was probably right, but her suggestion terrified me. So I called the couple in Queens and set up an interview.

I remained calm during the hour drive to Queens, the familiarity of Dad's little Buick grounding me. But as soon as I neared the address scribbled on my notebook paper, I began to shake. What the hell was I doing asking for a job? I knew absolutely nothing about dog and cat medicine. Nothing.

I found a parking spot by a meter under the El Train and snuck past the couples' storefront entrance a couple of times before finding the courage to enter. I glanced in the front window from the corner of my eye. The only person in the waiting room was a young woman sitting behind a desk. The third time, I exhaled, pulled open the door, and stepped in.

The girl looked up.

"I'm here for an interview." My voice croaked and, and of course, my right Eustachian tube closed.

"They're waiting for you. Have a seat. I'll let the doctors know you're here." She smiled.

A couple of minutes later, the office door opened and a short, red-headed woman wearing a white lab coat gestured for me to follow her to the back. A man, apparently her husband and partner, sat in a torn swivel chair in a crowded, book-lined alcove. When he stood up to shake my hand, his pants fell below his paunch. That, along with his frayed trousers and worn out sneakers, led me to believe that expectations couldn't be too high.

The well-manicured woman shot him a look. "Pull up your pants; you look like a slob."

Ouch! Criticizing her own husband in front of me? She could be trouble.

Forty-five minutes later it was official. They hired me as a vet tech! I'd start on Monday. From 8 a.m. to noon we'd see clients. Surgeries were scheduled from noon to two. Then a four-hour break, Italian-style, so they could go home for a big meal and nap. Evening appointments ran from 6 to 8 p.m., with clean-up after that. Hopefully I'd finish by 8:30 p.m. Six days a week. Pay just over minimum wage.

I drove two hours in traffic back to Lido, thrilled to share the good news with Mom.

Mom looked at me, incredulous, as I detailed my schedule. "You'll be driving two to four hours a day, depending on traffic. You probably won't be home till ten at night. And what are you going to do for the four hours your bosses are home eating and relaxing?"

"I'll study in the car."

"You're nuts," Mom said. "All this for five dollars an hour?"

"$5.50." I'd do it for free. My goal was to learn enough to pass the New York boards.

At 5 a.m. on Monday, Mom knocked on my door, per my instructions. I figured the trip could take over two hours with rush-hour traffic. I gulped down three cups of instant Taster's Choice and inhaled an English muffin with melted cheddar cheese and headed out.

Two and a half hours later, I arrived. Maria, the receptionist, buzzed me in. The Joneses welcomed me with a surprise. They'd gotten a small, black name tag with my name engraved in white: Marcie Fallek, DVM.

Chapter 12

DIY Doctoring

I tailed my bosses through morning appointments, eager to put my best foot forward. I jumped to clean the exam table with disinfectant and dry it off with paper towels, just as they'd shown me. I learned to draw up vaccines for the mostly Rottweiler and pit bull puppies that we saw throughout the morning. I listened closely to the doctors' conversations with clients, jotting stuff down in a small spiral notebook I carried. Mostly, my bosses rattled on about apparently basic stuff—heartworm disease and fleas and ticks and other parasites. I made sure to take good notes that first week, because I hadn't learned any of this in Italy.

Ralph, the husband, showed me how to tie a noose-like plastic leash into a figure eight around the hooks on the walled-side of a stainless-steel table. That was for the Rottweilers, which scared me. I'd never seen one prior to working there. Rottweilers were smart. Even the eight-week-old puppies looked me right in the eye as I tied them up.

"Make sure you tie the head real tight," Ralph said. That was good advice, as after the vaccines, when I loosened the lead, they whipped their heads around and lunged straight for me. I'd jump away just in time.

I overheard Elizabeth, the wife, tell her husband during a break, "I think we should get a Rottweiler. It'll be good protection." I can't say I blamed her. They lived nearby in what looked like a rough neighborhood, judging from the clients and the crowded, run-down store fronts.

Prior to my interview with the Joneses, I'd visited a veterinary hospital in the area where another Italian-trained vet worked. Dr. Luongo seemed bright and down-to-earth. I'd planned on asking him if he needed help. That is, until he pointed out a Doberman pinscher lying in a metal cage in the treatment room. "See that dog?" he said. "That's one of John Gotti's dogs. Gotti rescues dogs and brings 'em to me so I can find them homes. Somehow, that dog broke its leg here—I have no idea how. Now I gotta euthanize her. My neck is gonna be like his leg, if Gotti finds out." Despite my unhealthy fascination with the Mafia, I thought it best not to deal with the likes of John Gotti.

Back at the Joneses, my trouble began a week in, at surgery time. Ralph held a medium-sized terrier on the stainless-steel treatment table, and Elizabeth handed me a syringe. "Draw some blood," she ordered.

My heart stopped cold and sweat beaded in the small of my back. "I've never taken blood before," I admitted. I could barely hear myself speak.

"Watch. I'll take blood from the right leg first," Elizabeth said.

I watched, my temples throbbing.

Ralph swung into position and held the dog close, with his left arm, like in a hug, and put his right hand under the dog's front leg.

"Ralph is holding off the vein. Can you see the *cephalic* vein? If you can't see it, feel for it."

I saw nothing but a hairy leg.

Elizabeth said, "Wet the hair with alcohol, and hold the syringe in your right hand, like so. Then slide the needle into the vein and draw back." Elizabeth held a small piece of cotton on the leg as she removed the needle. She moved aside to make room for me.

Ralph shifted to the other side of the dog and hugged.

Elizabeth handed me a second syringe.

I felt like I was underwater. I took the dog's paw in my left hand and with the syringe clenched in my right, aimed it in the general direction of the vein.

About six inches away, I stopped. My hand started shaking like crazy, worse than Parkinson's. My step-grandfather had it, so I knew. A wave of anxiety swept through me, and my whole body buzzed.

"Why are you shaking?" Elizabeth demanded. "Stop shaking!"

I willed my hand to stop with all the mental force I could muster. But I shook even more. I could feel Elizabeth's eyes boring into my back.

Ralph released his stranglehold, and Elizabeth rolled her eyes. "I might have to send you to the shelter to learn venipuncture, like I sent Ralph."

(Later, I asked Ralph about this. He told me that because he'd had trouble hitting veins, Elizabeth had made him to go to the local animal pound to practice. Shelters need vets to euthanize unwanted dogs. This entailed injecting pentobarbital into their cephalic vein. Because the Queens kill shelter was packed, after just a couple of months Ralph had become an expert.)

Elizabeth called me over to the sink. She pointed to a big bottle filled with green liquid. "Fill the spray bottles with this disinfectant."

With Elizabeth and Ralph peering over my shoulder, I tried to pour disinfectant into the narrow-necked bottles. My hand shook like it had with the syringe. I didn't know what was happening. My hand never shook. And now, my whole body trembled. I turned toward them, my face twisted into an apologetic grimace. They stared some more, whispered to each other, then turned and disappeared into the surgery room with the dog.

Overwhelmed with shame and humiliation, I snuck past Maria, left the clinic, and crept into the back seat of my Dad's car, where I broke down in tears.

Who was I kidding? I'd never be a vet.

I stayed crouched low and peeked out every few minutes, until I saw the vets leave for break time. I couldn't study. Instead, I flung my book about laboratory animals onto the passenger seat and lay in a catatonic state for a few hours.

Elizabeth and Ralph had told me that they returned each evening at six, but I didn't know for sure. At 5:15 I peered out the window, looking right then left. With no sign of them, I slid out of the car, locked it, and hurried over to the corner deli. I bought a coffee, no sugar with 2-percent milk, and a Swiss cheese on rye. I peered around the corner in between gulps. At 5:45, I entered the waiting room, book in hand, and pretended to study. Ten minutes later, my bosses walked in. All business, they gestured to me to follow them back into the treatment area.

"We have a busy afternoon," Elizabeth said. "Make sure you clean the table after each patient." I managed a weak nod. They didn't say a word about the morning, and I sent a short prayer of thanks heavenward.

The first appointment of the evening was a pit bull puppy's recheck. It seemed my bosses had cropped its ears the week before. A tattooed guy with biceps like small melons, who looked like he couldn't wait to use them, cradled the dog.

"Hey man, Diego's ears are too short. He don't look like the other dogs."

The guy was right; to me, the dog looked earless.

Ralph glanced at the dog's ears. "That's the military cut," he said. "It's the new style: the vicious look." I'd never heard of the military cut, and I asked Ralph about it later.

"I made a mistake," he shrugged. "I cut one of the ears too short, so I had to even them out."

I later learned that our hospital had built a reputation for ear cropping. It seemed that many vets wouldn't cut ears, and in time I saw why: the surgery is tedious and bloody. Elizabeth or Ralph would first have to fit the dog's ears into a breed-appropriate stainless-steel mold, sort of like a cookie cutter. They'd tighten the screws and then cut along the edge. Ears are very vascular—they have tons of blood vessels—so the vets would have to stitch together the edges, like sewing a hem, something I had no patience for. Some vets refused to cut ears because it was so cruel. I knew that if I ever made it in this business I'd be in this camp.

The next patient of the evening was a limping German Shepherd, dirty and greasy and smelling of gasoline. When I reached over to pet the big guy, Rocky whipped his head around and went straight for my hand. He got me! The owner, who looked and smelled more or less like his dog, seemed amused.

"He's not used to petting. He's a guard dog. We keep him at the gas station. You know, to keep out the bad guys."

I stared at the hole in my finger. Elizabeth handed me a Band-Aid.

Next came a litter of what looked like little black rats. The animals lay listless in a filthy cardboard box. The kid who'd brought them told my boss that they'd stopped nursing. The kid didn't look like the nurturing type; he struck me more as the leader of a street gang. Elizabeth examined the creatures and discovered that they were puppies with infected tail stumps. Eventually the kid admitted he'd cut their tails off with scissors. I tried to hide my shock.

"The mother is a pure Rottweiler," the kid boasted. He didn't know what the father was. We sent the puppies home with oral antibiotics and ointment for the stumps. After the little hoodlum left, Elizabeth told me that some dog owners cut the tails themselves either because they want to sell the dogs as purebreds when they're not (and intact tails would thwart the ruse), or they want to save money.

Next we saw a schnauzer with diarrhea. The dog had probably gotten into some garbage. My boss gave the dog a couple of shots and dispensed antibiotics to be given at home. A few routine exams and vaccines filled the rest of the evening.

By the time appointments finished at 8:30 p.m., I was mentally exhausted and couldn't wait to leave. I'd have an hour or more drive to Lido and had to be back to the hospital by 8 a.m. As I reached for my jacket, Elizabeth handed me a mop and big metal pail. "Start in the surgery room and work your way forward. Finish with the waiting area."

The mop was heavy with long, white, stringy threads, the kind the janitor in my elementary school had used. I'd never mopped in my life. Our family cleaning woman used some kind of electric machine, and I'd washed my floors in Italy with a spray bottle and paper towels.

Elizabeth noticed my confusion. She demonstrated how to soak the mop in the larger compartment of the pail and squeeze out the excess liquid through the filter. "Make sure you rinse often. Otherwise you're just spreading the dirty water around." She turned on her heel to join her husband in the treatment room. I overheard them counting the day's stash—mostly cash. They sounded giddy.

The mop helped to steady my hands for the first time all day. This was something new I *could* do. And something I enjoyed. I loved to clean. As soon as I'd finished one of my fifty-one exams in Italy, I'd spend the whole next day cleaning my apartment, taking each and every book out of the bookcase, dusting each shelf as I listened to my sixties cassettes on my portable player. I don't know which gave me more joy, passing the exam or cleaning to music.

It was 11 p.m. by the time I got home. Mom waited up for me. She'd worried about me driving home so late at night from Queens. She set down a heaping plate of vegetarian chili at the full place setting waiting for me at our round Formica kitchen table. Too tired to answer her questions about my day, I gobbled down the food and asked if she could wake me at five.

A week later, despite my shaking hands—which only seemed to worsen— my bosses felt it was time for me to learn some surgery. After morning appointments, they pulled a black male cat out of a cage. Elizabeth's eyes pierced mine.

"We're going to castrate this cat," she said.

Chapter 13

Castration to CATastrophy

My empty hands shook, and I started to hyperventilate, but Elizabeth wasn't fazed.

"First, we have to anesthetize him." Elizabeth said. "Ralph is going to stretch the cat so you can inject the anesthesia into his femoral vein."

Ralph grabbed the cat by its scruff with one hand and gripped its back legs with the other, stretching the cat out like an accordion. The cat's eyes bugged out like a dead fish, but he couldn't move—which was the whole point, apparently, as this way he couldn't scratch or bite us. With her fingers, Elizabeth plucked out some hair from the inside of the cat's thigh and poured alcohol on it. "Now you can see the vein. Take that syringe and inject the ketamine in it."

I could barely make out the delicate blue line, my target. I steadied my right hand with my left and approached the cat. I managed to stick the needle in the leg, but apparently not in the vein. The cat screeched. (This is how I learned that ketamine burns if it gets outside of the vein.) The cat's skin swelled up into a big blue blob. I tried not to cry.

Elizabeth gave Ralph *the look*. He flipped the poor kitty onto its other side. Elizabeth repeated the plucking and wetting, and this time *she* injected the cat with the ketamine. Now the cat lay rigid and immobile, eyes wide open, staring at nothing. Elizabeth squeezed some antibiotic ointment into the cat's eyes, to prevent them from drying out. (Another thing I learned: Cats don't blink when they're anesthetized. It looks freaky if you're not used to it!)

"If you can tie a shoelace, you can castrate a cat," Elizabeth assured me. "I'll do one testicle, then you do the other."

"Even my seven-year-old son can do it," Ralph added.

Wait. Had Ralph just told me that his seven-year-old son castrated cats?

Elizabeth plucked fur from the scrotum and then held the testicle firmly in her hand. "Keep your thumb on one side of the ball and your index finger on the other. Cut through the skin with the scalpel, but not too deep. Then squeeze."

I watched as a naked testicle popped out, like a grape squeezed from its skin.

"Peel the epididymis from the testes," she said, explaining as she went along, as I stood there gawking. "Now you'll have the ball in your right hand and the epididymis in your left. Pretend you are tying your shoelace. Make a triple knot and pull tight."

I slowly approached the cat, which was lying on the grill of the dentistry table. Elizabeth and Ralph stood right behind me. I plucked hair from the other testicle, avoiding those open eyes. Then I took up a scalpel for the first time and made tiny baby cuts into the scrotum.

"Not like that," Elizabeth directed. "You're traumatizing the skin. Make one firm cut."

Somehow, I did it! I popped the testicle out of the scrotum and, despite my shaking hands, managed to push it through the hole three times. Then I tightened the knot.

"Use those sterile scissors and cut off the ball," Elizabeth said, eyeing my work. "Now stuff the knot into the scrotum and make sure none of it sticks out of the skin."

The surgery didn't require even one suture. A seven-year-old could totally do this. (And probably better than me. Their hands wouldn't shake.)

I looked forward to mopping.

Over the next few weeks we settled into a routine. I restrained the dogs and cats while my bosses drew blood, inserted IV catheters, and performed all the other procedures. The doctors did appreciate my work ethic, they told me so, but they worried about my shaking. I couldn't believe they didn't fire me for it.

One day a woman brought in her fourteen-year-old male tiger cat. "Muffin has been straining in his box lately," she told us. "He didn't eat today."

The scrawny cat with the matted coat lay listless on the table. It looked like he hadn't eaten in weeks.

Elizabeth frowned and pursed her lips as she felt the cat's abdomen. "Muffin is blocked," she said. "His bladder is huge—he probably hasn't urinated in three days." Elizabeth explained that this was a very serious condition. She began to squeeze the cat's bladder. A thin stream of urine dribbled out.

"Crystals can form in the bladder," she continued. "In a male cat it's dangerous, because they can block the cat's urethra so he can't pass urine. We need to admit Muffin immediately into the hospital. We'll have to catheterize him and keep him on IV fluids for three days to flush the toxins out of his bloodstream. He'll need careful monitoring along with antibiotics and antispasmodics."

I scribbled furiously in my notebook about this blocking thing—I'd never heard of it. When she released the cat's bladder to write up the estimate for treatment, I decided to pick up where she left off. I wanted to feel the bladder for myself, plus I wanted to be useful—I felt dumb standing idly by. I put my hand between the cat's hind legs and felt an enormous balloon. I began to squeeze the way Elizabeth had. Then my thumb slipped. Suddenly there was no more bladder. I watched in horror as the cat started to retch.

I stared wide-eyed and kicked Elizabeth under the table. She looked up from her writing. I nodded frantically, signaling a crisis. Oh my God, did I just kill the cat? I felt like I'd stepped into an empty elevator shaft.

I followed Elizabeth into the surgery. "I think I just broke the cat's bladder," I said. "I think he's dying!"

Expressionless, Elizabeth nodded calmly and motioned me back to the exam room, where the cat lay heaving on the stainless-steel table.

"Mrs. C., your cat is almost fifteen," Elizabeth declared, not missing a beat. "The prognosis is grim, given his age and overall condition. He's in bad shape. I've rethought the situation. I think it's more humane to euthanize him."

The woman burst into tears. She bent down and hovered over Muffin's face. "I'm so sorry my little Muffy!" she bawled.

Frozen with guilt and fear, I avoided Mrs. C's eyes. She signed the euthanasia agreement, still sobbing, and went out front to Maria to pay the bill. Elizabeth picked up the dying cat and disappeared into surgery. I followed her.

"What if she didn't want to put the cat to sleep?" I whispered.

"We could've admitted the cat and surgically repaired the bladder. But the cat *is* in bad shape. And this is more humane."

I felt terrible—for the cat and the owner. I tried but couldn't process the grief I'd just caused. Self-preservation kicked in. Could I lose my license? I still didn't have one to lose. Could she sue me? I didn't think so. Elizabeth covered for me, for which I was eternally grateful. Still, I felt I deserved some kind of karmic punishment. Maybe not an eye for an eye, but *something*.

I forced myself onward. Each time I recalled the retching cat, my mind froze, and I floated out of my body. I avoided handling the patients as much as possible.

In the meantime, Joe's stack of notes lay untouched. Mom had been right about that also: these fifteen-hour days exhausted me.

One day, I asked Elizabeth and Ralph if we could discuss my schedule. After surgery, we met up in the waiting room. I explained that with my heavy work schedule, I had no time to study for the boards. "I'd like to leave after surgery, so that I have the afternoon and evening to study." I paused, nervous. "I'll work for no pay," I added, hoping that that would clinch the deal.

"We need to discuss this. Could you wait here a few minutes?" They disappeared into the back and returned almost immediately. "Our only concern is that if we don't pay you, you won't work as hard." I assured them that wouldn't happen.

Did they really think I was doing this for the money?

When my fifteen-hour day was cut in half, I felt as if I'd been let out of prison.

Mom suggested that I study in her sewing room, an alcove off of her master bedroom, as school was out for the summer. This sounded good to me. I could spread my books and papers all over the carpet and recite out loud to my heart's content without disturbing my sister.

Still, after my parents went on vacation, all hell broke loose. Debra nagged me day and night. I dragged my mattress into the sewing alcove to minimize any contact, but it didn't help.

I struggled to see a way out. I couldn't afford an apartment of my own. I couldn't work a full-time job and also study for the boards. Plus, soon I'd have to start paying back my student loan at $450 a month.

One afternoon I sank to my knees and called out in desperation: "God, please help me!"

I lay sobbing on the blue carpet in Mom's bedroom when the telephone rang.

Chapter 14

Chop Chops and Veal Chops

An unfamiliar male voice greeted me. "Marcie?"

"Who's this?"

"Andy Cohen, from Manhattan. We met at the Connecticut test, in Hartford. Remember?"

No.

"I graduated from Italy too," he said.

I scanned my memory, but couldn't place the name or the voice.

He continued, "So, this morning a client asked me if I knew a cat-sitter. The guy's going away for the month of September to work on the Jerry Lewis Telethon. Your name popped into my head. He lives on West End Avenue and has one cat."

That got my attention. I imagined a beautiful prewar building overlooking the Hudson River.

"And, if you're looking, I can offer you a part-time job at my hospital," said the voice of a guy I couldn't place.

Five minutes prior, I'd seen no way out. Now some stranger was willing to pay me to stay in a beautiful apartment in my favorite part of Manhattan to watch his cat, and some other guy was offering me a job at his veterinary hospital. Plus, Andy said he could connect me with study partners for the boards.

He asked if I'd meet him for lunch the following week.

When the day arrived, I dressed in my Bologna best—long flowing skirt and high-heeled boots—stuff Italian girls wore to class in Italy. Trendy and funky. Perfect, I thought, for the Upper West Side.

I loved walking the city. I got off the train and floated seventy blocks up Seventh Avenue. As I made my way through the theater district, I drank in the names of shows on the marquees and soaked up the energy. I passed my favorite spot, Lincoln Center, with its big piazza and outdoor cafes. Not quite Europe, but not Lido Beach, and certainly not Queens.

At the hospital, I entered a packed waiting room and introduced myself to the receptionist, a mousy looking woman sitting behind a big desk. She told me the doctor would be out shortly.

I sat on a bench along the wall and took in the scene. The clients looked like me—Jewish, curly hair, hippy-looking, and as I listened to their conversations, I realized they sounded like me—New York accent, loud, opinionated, probably liberal. My people, my tribe. And my kind of dogs, cute fluffy ones: golden retrievers, spaniels, mutts. Not a single vicious-looking dog in sight!

When a thin, scruffy, bearded man in a lab coat entered the waiting room, I recognized him immediately. He was the guy I'd breakfasted with the morning before the Clinical Competency test. Like most of the examinees, I'd traveled from out of town and stayed at the conference center/hotel to be ready for the early morning start of the exam. At breakfast, a fellow graduate from Bologna had recognized me and called me over to join him and the scruffy guy and some others for breakfast. Andy was halfway through a huge plate of eggs, bacon, and toast, with, I think, pancakes on the side. My stomach fluttered with anticipation so I could only pick at my muffin. I had to ask, "How can you eat so much? Aren't you nervous?"

Andy explained between mouthfuls that the last time he'd taken the test, he hadn't eaten enough for breakfast and was starving by noon. "I ate so much at lunch that I fell asleep during the afternoon test and didn't finish it."

Now, at the hospital, I rose to greet him.

"We're meeting my associate at a Chinese restaurant down the block. I'll show you around the hospital afterward," he said, without even a smile.

It seemed like all eyes followed us to the door. As we threaded our way down the crowded sidewalk toward the restaurant, he filled me in on his practice and, in short order, we reached the restaurant. No white tablecloths, but a decent enough place with one of those glassed-in outdoor dining areas, my favorite for people-watching. "Your friend is waiting for you," the maître d' said, pointing us in that direction.

A heavily made-up bleached blonde watched us from her table for four. I recognized her immediately: Gail! My ex-best friend from Bologna, the one who'd stolen my boyfriend, Tuvia! The one Baba knew had broken my heart. After our breakup, Tuvia had moved in with Gail in the apartment directly above mine for two years until he dumped her. Then Gail had come crying to me. For sympathy! I'd actually felt sorry for her at the time.

Anyhow, that was ancient history, almost ten years ago. Now she worked for Andy? What were the odds?

I fought an impulse to bolt from the restaurant. Gail glanced at me, her blue eyes cold, and then she turned to Andy. "You're late," she snapped.

Who speaks like that to a boss?

Andy ordered a three-course meal, while Gail and I picked at a couple of appetizers. When the bill came, Andy mentioned that he'd forgotten his wallet. Gail shot him a scathing look as she pulled out her credit card. "Very convenient. You *always* forget your wallet. You invited *me* to lunch."

Andy suddenly remembered an appointment with a VIP client. He asked if I minded forgoing the hospital tour for now. But he hired me on the spot. I told him to give the Jerry Lewis Telethon guy my number. Before he left, Andy added that he could get me as many pet-sitting jobs as I wanted. "People want a sitter they can trust. You can't get better than a vet," he said. I'd never thought of that. I figured they'd want experience, and I'd never pet-sat before.

I had landed a job and a place to live. I rushed out of the restaurant and searched for a pay phone. I called Grandma and asked if I could stay with her between house-sitting gigs. I couldn't co-exist in a ten-room house with my family, but my grandmother and I thrived in her L-shaped studio.

Grandma's voice lit up when she heard the news. What foods should she buy me? She knew that I didn't eat meat, and she wanted to make sure I wouldn't go hungry. As if one could go hungry living near restaurant row—55th Street—along with the convenient little grocery store across the street, Ernest Klein and Company, which Grandma called Tiffany's. I told her just to make sure she had real milk for my coffee. I couldn't stand the liquid creamer that she and my parents swilled.

I quit my job in Queens, giving them two-week notice. They didn't seem to mind. I packed my clothes, my books, and my notes and shed no tears as I left Lido Beach.

I settled into the telethon producer's cavernous three-bedroom apartment in a stately prewar building on West End Avenue, feeling right at home. Maybe this area was in my DNA. Mom had grown up with Grandma and Grandpa on West End Avenue, just a few blocks away! In fact, she was voted Miss West End Avenue in high school, she'd once told me. My father and his family had lived close by, at the Bel Nord (the sister building of the famed Dakota) which took up a full city block on 86th Street, between Amsterdam and Columbus. The place looked like Buckingham Palace, with its magnificent black and gold gates, high archways built to accommodate horse and carriage, guardhouse, and gardened courtyard. When Nana, Aunt Carole, and Aunt Irene had left their ten-room, $200 per month, rent-controlled apartment in the 1970s to relocate to God's-waiting-room, Miami, it broke my heart.

Oliver, the producer's orange tabby, made the perfect roommate. He didn't make noise, minded his business, and cuddled often.

The first day I set off for Dr. Andy's hospital, I felt I was exactly where I was supposed to be as I bustled up Broadway, rivulets of energy running up and down my body, blending in with the locals racing to work. Feeling very New York, I grabbed a coffee and croissant from a take-out place.

I reached the hospital's packed waiting room in fifteen minutes. Once inside, I heard a commotion and checked for the source. Dr. Andy was fawning over a pretty young woman sitting by the receptionist's desk that I recognized as a famous news anchor.

Dr. Andy asked me to follow him into the back. His office was little more than a closet, crowded with books and junk and a desk loaded with stacks of papers. The mess calmed my nerves—maybe expectations wouldn't be too high, like at the Joneses.

Andy showed me the notes he was working on for the National Boards, which he still hadn't passed, and then took me on a tour of the hospital. He treated me as a colleague, with respect. In the back, a huge, swarthy guy with slicked-down hair introduced himself to me. His name was Paco and apparently, he had just wrapped up an operation. He transferred a cigarette from the thick fingers of his right hand to his left, to hug me. "Welcome!" he said, with some kind of accent.

At the hospital, I worked as a tech, as I hadn't yet taken my New York boards. Andy wasn't allowed to see clients because he still hadn't passed anything. Paco hid in the back, away from prying eyes, doing the surgeries. I learned that he was what vets called a "chop-chop": a vet from a foreign country, in his case Peru, who hadn't been or couldn't be licensed in America. Gail was the only one licensed to see clients. Now I understood how she could get away with her nonsense.

On my first day, as Gail was about to enter one of the exam rooms, Andy said, "Why don't you go in with her?"

Seeing little choice, I trailed her into a small, glassed-in room. A bawling woman hovered over a motionless white cat on a stainless-steel exam table. Apparently, the appointment was for euthanasia. Gail ignored the woman and the cat and turned toward me with a self-satisfied smile. Placing her hands on her buttocks, she began to plié.

"Remember how Luigi said that if we had good technique, our butt cheeks would be firm and round like two *ciliegi* (cherries)?" We'd attended ballet class together years ago in Bologna. I wasn't sure if she was trying to impress me or the client, but we both looked at Gail in astonishment.

At the end of my first week, I confessed my insecurity around anything scalpel to Paco. He wrapped a sweaty arm around me. "Don't worry. Paco show you everything. You be fine." He was true to his word: He showed me—and Andy—how to do everything.

I hung out with Shelley, the receptionist, during slow times. It seemed the non-veterinarians who worked in these hospitals were the true animal-lovers. I asked Shelley about the gold-framed photo on her desk: five cats sitting in a circle in front of five ceramic food bowls, each bowl on an individual placemat. "That's my family," she said with a proud smile. Shelley must have been in her mid-forties, unmarried, no children. She seemed happy. I worried that this would be me in ten years. I wanted a partner and children.

When my West End Avenue housesitting job ended, I packed up and took a cab to Grandma's. I had another two weeks before my next job as a pet-sitter.

"You must be starving," she said as she opened the door. I dumped my suitcase in the dining area and kissed her cheek. "I'm so happy you're back from Italy." She beamed. "I've waited ten years for you. That's why I'm still alive!"

God bless that woman. I found it hard to reconcile that she and my mother were related. She oozed love and acceptance.

I took my seat at the dining-room table, and Grandma offered me veal chops. "I wish you'd eat one."

"Grandma, you know I don't eat meat."

My family harassed me for not eating meat. They thought I was part of some Indian cult. Though Grandma looked hurt, she served up my favorite frozen dinner: Stouffer's spinach soufflé. Grandma always kept it in the freezer for me, along with their macaroni and cheese.

I changed the subject. "Why don't we play Spite and Malice after dinner?" Grandma loved card games, and I loved to play cards with her; it forced me to relax, when, normally, I programmed every minute of my life.

"Where would you like to eat tomorrow night?" she said, happy again. "I want to take you somewhere special."

"Can't we just eat here and make blintzes or something?" Although I didn't vomit anymore, I thought about food all the time—what I didn't eat, what I wouldn't eat, what I could eat. With a mind so filled with thoughts of food, I couldn't bear more coming at me. "You're always talking about food. You know I can't stand that."

Her face fell. "I never have anyone to eat out with."

"Oh, all right. Let's eat wherever you want."

"Would you like French or Italian?"

"French." I knew the place—I loved their cheese fondue.

After our card game, I followed Grandma into her bedroom alcove. Seven p.m.—time for *The McNeil Lehrer Report*. She turned on the TV to channel 13, PBS, and sank into her blue velvet armchair. I sat beside her on the two-toned blue shag carpet. She smiled at me and repeated what she always said at 7 p.m.: "Time to listen to some smart people."

At eight, when the show ended, Grandma kissed me goodnight and climbed into her twin bed in the alcove and was snoring away within minutes. I made up the couch with the sheets and blankets she'd left out. I propped my picture of Sai Baba on the marble coffee table and wrapped the *japamala* around my fingers. Filled with gratitude, I looked deep into the eyes of the photo. *Thank you so much for everything.*

Chapter 15

Bovine, 'er Divine, Intervention

My confidence grew as the weeks flew by. With Paco's encouragement, I drew blood, inserted IV catheters, and assisted with minor surgical procedures, such as cat castrations, abscesses, and lacerations. My hands didn't shake once.

I pet-sat in the most incredible spaces. Each time I crossed the threshold of a new apartment, I entered another fascinating life. On the bedroom wall of one apartment, I saw several blown-up photos of a familiar face. Once I'd deciphered the dedications, I realized I was sleeping in the bed of Sigmund Freud's niece! As with many New Yorkers who were crazy about their animals, she was also a bit crazy. She, like all the others, had left numerous pages of instructions, either handwritten or typed. She spelled out the route where I should walk the dogs and counselled me to beware of the bagel bakery where "the girls" would "beg shamelessly" for handouts.

I followed all directions to a T.

But when one woman wrote in her five-page, single-spaced instructions to lie on my left side on the couch and make soft cooing noises, so that the cats would curl up and sleep under my right arm, I drew the line. I fed the cats, then I slept in my bed and they slept in theirs.

I tried to study with Andy, my boss, but it was a waste of time. I knew more than he did. Just like in Italy, I never realized how much I knew until I compared myself to others.

I studied alone for the New York boards every single day, either at my house-sitting jobs or at Grandma's. In my clients' apartments, I'd spread my books and notes on the floor or bed and recite out loud, disturbing no one—the dogs and cats didn't mind. At the Carnegie House, I'd sit at the dining room table, while Grandma, in her blue velvet chair, would read a library book so as not to disturb me with the TV. She didn't seem to mind listening to me recite, and she whispered if she spoke on the phone. With Grandma's love surrounding me, I felt invincible and like I could accomplish anything. She told me I was second to no one.

When the University of Pennsylvania weekend prep course rolled around in May, I took the Long Island Railroad back to Lido, where Joe and his friend Chuck collected me. They felt like the big brothers I'd read about in *Seventeen Magazine*, the ones I'd always wished I had. I knew I could trust them. Joe was a happily married gentleman and Chuck a Mormon who wouldn't even drink Coca Cola. We shared a motel room and, miracle of miracles, I was able to fall asleep on my pull-away mattress nestled into the far corner.

The teachers at UPenn shoved a staggering amount of material at us. I hoped Joe was right, that these two days would suffice to pass the New York State Boards.

On the drive home, Joe urged me to take the test with him and Chuck in June and not wait another six months.

"Are you crazy? I'm nowhere near ready," I said. I figured I'd need at least a year more to prepare.

"Don't worry, it's like Italy. You don't have to know everything. If you fail, you can take it again."

I shuddered.

"Take a chance," he urged. "At the very least, you'll learn what they want. Plus, you know more than you think."

I was terrified to waste one of my three opportunities, but heeded Joe's advice and registered.

A month later, the three of us drove to Cornell to take the boards, with Joe, again, at the wheel. This time I got my own hotel room. I wasn't the least bit nervous because I knew I was going to fail. I fell asleep quickly and, well-rested, met up with everyone in the morning. I watched, detached, as the other veterinarians crammed.

The proctors handed out our schedules. My first station was Equine. I found the designated area and waited outside the barn with eleven other vets.

Come my turn, I entered a large dirt pen and met my examiner and a horse. First question: "How much does this horse weigh, Dr. Fallek?"

I'd spent so many years dieting and standing on scales. I gave my best guess.

"1400 pounds?"

Somehow, I guessed correctly.

"Please pick up the horse's hoof and show me where the 'frog' is."

Of course, I knew where the frog was: that hard, black, V-shaped thing on the bottom of the foot. Although I'd never owned a horse, I'd been riding since I was seven. And all I'd ever wanted was a horse. At UPenn, I'd learned how to lift the foot. I pointed to the frog. In fact, I answered all the examiner's questions correctly.

The next guy grilled me on laboratory animals, rodents and other things that researchers experiment on. I'd heard horror stories about this section of the Boards. One friend of mine, a graduate from Bologna, hadn't known how to pick up a rabbit during her exam. I didn't know either—I only knew that you had to be careful. If they struggle, they can break their back. In my friend's case, the rabbit had jumped out of the cage and hopped down the hallway, with Laurie and the proctor running after it. She failed.

The examiner directed me to a cage with a calico creature that looked like a bloated mouse on steroids. I recognized the critter—a guinea pig. I sighed in relief. They're gentle and easy to handle. I'd studied the guinea pig from a paperback green spiral book on lab animals for vet techs that I'd found at Barnes & Noble. Guinea pigs were easy, with only a few salient facts to learn. The thing I remembered most is that they are sensitive to antibiotics, which can kill them.

The examiner asked me to name a few diseases. In my mind's eye, I saw the couple of pages from my book. Like people, and unlike dogs, guinea pigs don't make their own vitamin C and therefore, like us, can get scurvy. (Fun fact: It is because of their similarities with us that researchers use them for lots of medical experiments. That's how we got the term *guinea pig*.)

I rattled off some diarrheal and respiratory diseases. Next, the examiner asked me what made the guinea pig sometimes difficult to experiment on. I told him about the antibiotics.

Oh my God. I started to get nervous—I could actually have a shot at passing these boards after all.

The third station terrified me. Bovine. I could barely breathe as I waited my turn outside the room with the other examinees. When a vet candidate finished the exam, a minute or two elapsed before the next vet entered the hot seat. I overheard a guy who was leaving say something about a "ripe ovary in Box #3."

When my name was called, I stood in front of a row of five big wooden boxes that looked like those turn-of-the-century cameras, the kind with the drapes over them. They weren't cameras though. They were fake rectums, leading to fake uteri and fake ovaries. The examiner directed me to Box #3. He told me to put on a glove, put my arm through the hole in the box and describe the stage of the ovary and whether the cow was ready to be artificially inseminated. The idea was to simulate a rectal exam. Thanks to Divine intervention, the Herkimer farmer, and the comment from the last exiting student, I (a) knew how to put on the long-sleeved glove and (b) answered the question correctly.

I went to the barn for my second and third bovine questions. A vet (examiners were local veterinarians) stood in front of a pile of enormous metal instruments. He pointed to one and told me to identify it. I recognized this from the UPenn course. It looked like a giant nutcracker. "Emasculator!"

He showed me another instrument. "What is this used for?"

"To dehorn a calf."

"What anesthesia would you use?"

"A nerve-block."

Next station: pigs. No actual live pigs, thank God. I'd skipped studying swine husbandry and had only glossed over pig diseases. As the twelve of us gathered outside, I felt like a horse at the starting gate, ready to break for the best position. I knew there'd be twelve tables with twelve examiners. I may not have known much about pigs, but I'd learned an essential survival skill in Italy: how to read people—and I wanted the pick of the litter. When the door cracked open, I shot through and scanned the room. I raced to a smiling, elderly, plump farmer to my far right, avoiding the stern, thin woman with glasses straight ahead of me.

I took my seat. The pig vet smiled. "How long is the gestation period of the pig?"

"Three months?"

"You mean three months, three weeks, and three days, right?"

I nodded. He scribbled something in his notepad.

Second question: "What is the typical litter size of a domestic pig?"

"Ten?" I postulated.

"You mean twelve," said he, writing again on his clipboard.

The rest of the exam followed suit.

"You did it, Dr. Fallek!" He grinned.

Fifth station: small animals, dogs and cats. I guessed again and hoped that I guessed right.

Sixth and last station: the goat. I knew nothing about goats.

I entered a large barn and looked around. Each examiner held a goat on a short leash. I spotted a laid-back farmer-type on the near side of the arena, but I wasn't quick enough. Another woman got there first. *Oy vey.* I got stuck with a weedy, dour-faced man.

When the guy asked me my first question, I didn't have a clue.

What the hell was I doing here?

I chewed my lip, embarrassed and humiliated, and said nothing. I had nothing *to* say. With nary a glance in my direction, Dr. Goat slowly raised the clipboard, answer-side towards me. I tried not to look and focused my eyes on the goat. He positioned the clipboard so that it was directly in front of my face! After each question, he repeated this maneuver, and I didn't have to endure another moment's awkward silence.

Thank you, God.

Several weeks later, I received notice that I'd failed the bovine and small animal sections, and therefore, failed the New York State Boards.

Joe and Chuck also failed. Joe said we should drive back to Cornell to review our tests and hopefully find some grading errors that would allow us to contest the results. I couldn't imagine the New York State Board of

Veterinary Medical Examiners making any mistakes grading our tests. Besides, I didn't want to see how I'd screwed up. But Joe insisted, so I joined the boys on the road trip.

Joe and Chuck, along with all the other vets, came armed with piles of books, ready for battle. I went empty-handed.

We streamed into a spacious, sunlit room. An examiner handed me my test, along with the answer booklet. I looked around at the tense faces poring over the material. I strolled over to a tall bar-like chair at a lone table and placed my test answers on the left side of the table and the answer booklet on my right. I opened to page one. Halfway through the bovine section, I saw a mistake! A huge, glaring mistake. I had answered correctly! They'd graded me incorrectly! Adrenaline coursed through my body as my eyes darted between my test and the answer booklet. I found a second mistake and then a third. A couple of hours later, I handed in my papers.

Another miracle? It sure felt like it.

I'd have to wait several months to find out.

Chapter 16

Pass the Nutmeg

In the meantime, I learned I'd passed the Clinical Competency Test (the fun test), which, together with my high score on the National Boards, which I'd taken in the fall, licensed me in Connecticut! Since I hadn't yet heard from Albany regarding the status of my challenges to the New York State Boards, and I couldn't count on passing, I started my job search in Connecticut.

I'd always liked the "Nutmeg State." My family and I would often visit our cousins, the Martins, in Stamford. My cousin Nancy was exactly my age, so we'd hang out together growing up. Once, during college break, the two of us hacked a couple of horses in Greenwich for a trail ride. I considered myself a city girl, but as I settled into the saddle and drank in the pine-scented air of the woods, I felt right at home. "I would love to live here!" I shouted to Nancy. Oh, to be living the simple life in Greenwich with my horse.

Nancy halted her mare and twisted around to face me. "Marcie, do you know what it costs to live in Greenwich?" I did not. But from her tone, I guessed it was on par with Beverly Hills.

When I launched my job search, my mother called Nancy's mother, Shirley, to see if I could stay with them while I job-hunted.

The Martins gave me a key and told me the extra bedroom was mine as long as I needed it.

Shirley and George treated me like the family I'd only dreamed of. I'd spend a couple of hours each morning in my pajamas hanging out with Shirley at the breakfast table, talking love and life. When George came home from work, we'd drink wine together, comparing American and Italian vintages.

On the other hand, the day Nancy came for a visit, she admitted to me that her husband, Tony, had bet her ten dollars that I'd never graduate from vet school. I felt so hurt that I told my mother. Mom said, "Well, I made a $100,000 bet that you would." I'd never thought of that. My $20,000 student loan could never have covered the expenses generated in my ten years abroad. My parents had paid the difference.

Between breakfast coffee and evening wine, I scoured the American Veterinary Medical Association (AVMA) journal's classified section. Within a few weeks, I read of a job opening in Westport.

Westport! I'd visited Westport between my freshman and sophomore year of college, when I was auditioning to be someone's roommate. Freshman year, I'd studied at Emory University in Atlanta: But one year there had sufficed. While other American colleges were erupting in protests, the girls at Emory were voting to prohibit boys from our dorm rooms (to preserve our feminine mystique). Even though I was a virgin, who'd never even tried pot, the Dixie belles considered me a hippy because I wore jeans. I transferred to Boston University, the antidote, in my opinion, to the South.

I'd found a couple of potential roommates to share an apartment with, in Back Bay. Lisa was one of them. Her dad, a vice president of AT&T, had insisted on meeting the Fallek family before he'd allow the *shidduch* (match). Mom, Dad, and I drove to their home on Beachside Avenue in Westport.

As Dad drove our blue Oldsmobile through the electric-powered entry gate, past the two-story caretaker's cottage (bigger than our home), and down the winding driveway to the three-story Spanish-style mansion, I felt like a Beverly Hillbilly. Lisa's Mary Tyler Moore and Dick Van Dyke look-alike parents answered the door and ushered us into the foyer, just as Lisa exited the elevator (the elevator!) in cut-offs and flip-flops, munching on a shrimp. Somehow, we Falleks must have passed muster, as Lisa and I later roomed together.

That was fifteen years prior. Now, Westport meant Paul Newman! What girl wasn't in love with him? Every magazine article I'd read about him mentioned he lived in toney Westport. I couldn't believe little old me from Lido Beach could live in the same town as Paul Newman! My hands shook once again, as I dialed the number of the veterinary hospital in Westport.

Chapter 17

From Shabby to Chic

The following day, I chose my interview clothes carefully: trim, tan skirt with a long-sleeved, V-neck, yellow cotton shirt neatly tucked in. I even wore pointy beige flats and stockings.

As usual, I arrived way too early. Not wanting to appear overanxious, I hung out in my car until the appointed time and then whispered a brief, but heartfelt prayer. The waiting room was empty and the receptionist busy on the phone, which gave me time to scope out the place.

It looked different from any other hospital I'd seen. Blond wood walls and beige tiles welcomed clients, almost as if into someone's home. Forest-green cushioned-bench seating gave the place a Ralph Lauren look. No gray metal industrial bookcases stocked with flea and tick products, medicated shampoos, and other drugs for pets for sale. No advertisements for insecticides featuring dogs' hearts or intestines crawling with worms. Instead, framed posters of farm animals adorned the room. A delicate, wrought-iron baker's rack filled with animal paraphernalia rested against the wall.

It seemed that this veterinarian loved animals. Maybe she'd even be a vegetarian. Otherwise why would she have pictures of happy pigs and cows? Those animals sure didn't smile on factory farms or in slaughterhouses.

A red-haired girl at the desk called me over, and in a clipped British accent told me to take a seat. Too antsy to sit, I paced the room, checking out the artwork.

One poster caught my eye—a willowy woman in a Victorian dress. Three dogs lay at her feet, and four cats perched on her shoulder, all staring adoringly at her. I couldn't believe it: I had that same Steinlen Art Nouveau poster hanging on my bedroom wall in Lido Beach! Before leaving for vet school, I'd seen this poster for sale at my hairdresser's. It was expensive—twenty dollars—but I bought it anyway. It reminded me of Walt Disney's *The Three Lives of Thomasina,* a Sunday night TV movie that told the story of a young woman considered to be a witch by the townsfolk, who healed animals with love. The movie had touched my soul as a child and still resonated at twenty-three, when I'd bought the print. Healing with love. That was my dream.

I didn't take that poster to Bologna. Instead, I kept it on my wall in Lido for inspiration. Each time I returned home from Italy, I focused on the picture, envisioning myself as the lady in the long, flowing red dress surrounded by grateful animals. I told myself I would hang it in my office when, and only when, I became a vet.

Now, here I stood, twelve years later. It seemed I was exactly where I was supposed to be.

A slight, make-up-free woman, wearing slacks and a white lab coat, entered the room. She looked like me, but slimmer and with gray curly hair instead of my blonde. She approached in a slightly pigeon-toed way, hand extended.

"Hi. You must be Marcie. Glad to meet you. Let me show you around."

I followed Dr. Amy Russell into a spacious, sun-drenched exam room, fronted by a large bay window. Bright light filled the room and me with its cheery glow. Toenail scratches on the bare wooden bench seat suggested animal-friendliness. Framed canvases of dogs and cats hung on the walls—painted by her daughter, Amy said. A second, smaller exam room was also filled with tasteful animal art.

Dr. Russell led me into the treatment area, where she introduced me to the staff. Barbara and Susan, the two techs, smiled and welcomed me. Tess, the bubbly redhead at the desk, turned out to be Irish. All women. I loved it.

We climbed the stairs to Dr. Russell's private office. She complimented me on my appearance, sounding almost wistful. I didn't tell her I normally dressed like her: baggy pants and non-matching shirt, functional, not feminine. I wore make-up only for very special occasions, this being one of them.

I'd heard from a colleague that Dr. Russell had graduated from vet school later in life, just as I had. I could tell that she'd also entered veterinary medicine for the love of animals. She told me that she refused to crop ears and dock tails. She rescued animals, refusing to support pet stores or breeders. She was, indeed, a vegetarian. And despite her gray hair, refined taste, and understated clothing and decor, she was also a New York Jew.

The conversation flowed seamlessly into my responsibilities and duties. No question if, just when and how. I'd work seven days a week, 8 a.m. to 6 p.m. on Monday through Friday and half a day on Saturday. Sunday, no clients, but I'd be expected to treat the hospitalized animals Saturday afternoon and twice on Sunday.

I'd get every other major holiday off, five a year. No official sick days, but she'd pay half my health insurance, a practically unheard-of bonus in the vet world. No personal days. Five vacation days after one year of work.

"I do my own emergencies," Dr. Russell declared. "My clients deserve my continuous care."

I gasped inwardly; I'd sworn I'd never take a job that required emergency duty. If I thought my phone could ring in the middle of the night, I'd never fall asleep. Almost all veterinarians referred clients to an emergency hospital after hours. This could be a deal-breaker.

"Only until 10 p.m.," the doctor added after my pause. "After that, the emergency clinic will take over. I'll be available by phone if an emergency comes in that you feel you can't handle."

I accepted!

Wow, a real job in a real hospital. In Westport! In fact, I'd *have* to live in Westport, Dr. Russell said, to be close by for emergencies. I wasn't sure how I could afford it, but I loved the idea that I *had* to live in Paul Newman's town.

After I accepted, Dr. Russell said, "Let's discuss your salary."

I asked for $23,000, but I would have settled for $20,000.

"$25,000 a year," she stated.

Wow again! All those years of struggle and sacrifice would finally pay off. I signed a year-long contract and imagined a long and happy future together. I knew if I worked hard, I could make it work.

My parents drove up from Lido to help me apartment-hunt. We found a shabby realtor's office in a neighboring town that also did rentals. I told a frumpy middle-aged woman my price range—around $400 a month—and she said, "Difficult, but not impossible."

My take-home pay worked out to be about $1,700 a month. Though Mom had taught me that rent shouldn't exceed a quarter of one's take-home pay, that didn't allow for my student loan. The $450 a month I owed the government hung like a black cloud over my head.

We followed the agent to a ramshackle, peeling, wooden house. My parents and I looked at each other as we parked next to several beat-up cars in the dirt driveway. We walked up the rickety stairs to the main level. We looked around—four bedrooms for four roommates. I glanced at Mom. She looked revolted.

Dirty and old I could deal with, but when my insomnia started in vet school in Italy, I'd lived with only one roommate at a time, chosen primarily for their absence. I'd figure out during their interviews which candidates would spend most nights away—either at their parents' or boyfriend's house. I needed absolute quiet to sleep. I definitely couldn't live with three other people. If this was all I could afford, I'd have to decline the job.

I said no thanks to the rental and we headed back to my cousins', picking up a copy of the *Westport Minuteman*, the local newspaper, en route. An ad for a one-bedroom apartment in the center of town caught my eye. I set up an appointment with the landlord.

My parents and I met Bob, the landlord, in the parking lot of 165 Post Road East, in downtown Westport. The apartment was right above Haagen-Dazs. Oh my God. It would be like an alcoholic living above a liquor store. Even though I hadn't vomited since my sessions with Dr. Adams, ice cream was the one thing that challenged my bulimia. I peeked in the window. They had frozen yogurt also. Thank God, that I could manage.

While *shmoozing* with Bob, a grungy, hippy-looking type, my father poked and prodded and discovered that Bob was Jewish, from London. The reason he'd come to the United States was because he didn't get into the college of his choice, Cambridge University.

"So, where'd you go?" Dad asked.

"Harvard."

They loved him.

I followed Bob and my parents up a narrow stairwell into a spanking clean, newly carpeted, adorable three-hundred-square-foot apartment. A skylight brightened the living room, so you didn't notice there weren't any windows. The bedroom, no bigger than Grandma's alcove, could hold a single bed and a tiny dresser. But it would be all mine. Only catch: $800 a month.

Mom took me aside. "Take it. Don't tell Daddy that I will pay half the rent, and don't worry about your loan. I'll pay it off. The rest is on you."

My eyes filled with happy tears. I had arrived.

Chapter 18

"Mr. Newman in Room One"

I'd never seen clients by myself. I'd never diagnosed or treated diseases. I'd only performed surgeries that seven-year-olds could do. Mostly, I'd watched as other vets worked.

The idea of me and the client alone in the room together made me dizzy. The thought of making a mistake terrified me. I knew that I was a perfectionist. But with the well-being of someone's beloved pet, even its life, resting on my judgment, there was truly no room for error.

I trusted that Dr. Russell would be true to her word and help me. But just in case, I hid several small notebooks in a backpack on the rear stairwell. I figured if I was unsure of how to proceed, I could scurry to my notes before or during appointments to check the differential diagnoses and treatment protocols.

On Day One, while hanging out with the techs in the treatment area, Tess called me on the intercom: "Dr. Fallek, Mr. Paul Newman is waiting for you in Room One."

I thought I would faint! First, because she called me Dr. Fallek. Second, because it was Paul Newman. Paul Newman! How could Paul Newman be my very first client on my very first day as a licensed vet? How could I be alone in a room with Paul Newman? Especially, because I didn't know what the hell I was doing?

Terrified, I rushed upstairs to Dr. Russell's office. Breathless, I told her that Paul Newman was in the exam room and *begged* her to take over. She seemed unfazed. I trailed her downstairs and into the exam room, like a five-year-old following her mommy.

Mr. Newman stood on the far side of the stainless-steel exam table with a miniature schnauzer in his arms—the one I'd seen in ads for his charity on TV. I expected the sultry sexiness of the Paul Newman from *Cat on a Hot Tin Roof*, or the devilishly handsome Paul Newman, the one with the mischievous smile, chiseled features, and cleft chin from *Butch Cassidy and the Sundance Kid*. Instead, he looked rather ordinary—short and slight, gray-haired, with a receding hair line. If I didn't know it was Paul Newman, I wouldn't have taken a second look if he passed me on the street. Still, I could barely breathe and couldn't take my eyes off of him.

Amy stood between the near wall and the table. I stood in right field, mute and immobile, like I was role-playing in my veterinary gear: white coat, stethoscope, and nametag. I was close enough to watch, but far enough that Paul knew I wasn't in charge.

Amy asked Mr. Newman what was wrong with his dog.

"He hurt his paw." Mr. Newman frowned as he placed the dog on the table.

While Amy inspected the dog's foot and Paul looked on (were we on a first name basis now?), I stared at that famous face with those legendary blue eyes.

Amy straightened, a serious look on her face. "He broke his toenail above the quick," she said.

We'd never studied this in vet school. I quizzed myself. What would I do? I'd treat the dog's nail the way I'd treated my own if I had a hangnail. I would trim it as close to the break as possible. I would tell him that the rest would grow out or that he could come back in a couple of weeks and I'd snip it off. But that's not what Amy said. She told him the dog had to be hospitalized and anesthetized to cut the broken nail. The dog could be discharged late afternoon.

(Thank God I'd asked Dr. Amy to take over!)

Mr. Newman's celebrated eyes widened. "Can't you just cut the nail here in the room?"

Dr. Russell explained that cutting through the quick would be painful and bloody. She drew up an estimate.

Paul grimaced his consent, signed the hospital release form, and left.

I'd never imagined that cutting a broken nail would be such a big deal, with a bill in the hundreds. But I guessed she supposed that Paul Newman could afford it.

Paul Newman on Day One! I couldn't wait to see what would come next.

On Day Two, a smartly dressed middle-aged man stormed into the exam room with a six-month-old golden retriever puppy. He had come for a second opinion. Angry and worried, he lifted the dog's front legs.

Glaring at me, he pointed to his dog's genitals. "Look at this. Just look at this!"

Heart thumping, I stooped down and followed his finger. *Look at what?*

"Her recessed vulva! I want to know exactly what my options are and precisely how this will affect Sophie's long-term health."

I stared at him, speechless. I knew I didn't have any cheat sheets on recessed vulvas, so I hurried to the boss to ask her what the heck a recessed vulva was and what to do about it.

"I'll take care of it," she said.

Turns out, Sophie needed major surgery.

I'd never be prepared!

The next few weeks felt daunting, but between my notes on the stairwell and Amy's help, I managed.

Then Amy decided it was time for me to spay a cat. *Oy vey.* Cat spays are often the first real surgery a novice vet performs, because they are considered relatively easy. Amy had told me she'd felt insecure when she started performing surgery, which made me feel better. We women, full of insecurities, understood each other.

On a Tuesday, after morning appointments, my heart raced as I readied myself for the spay. Both Susan and Barbara had started prepping and preparing. If a crisis occurred, at least I wouldn't have to face it alone. Susan wiped down the metal operating table with an antiseptic solution, pulled the rolling instrument table next to the anesthesia machine, and placed a sealed sterile surgical pack on top of the table.

Amy had me follow her into the treatment area to prep for surgery. She stretched the cat, the same way Ralph from Queens had, and told me to inject the ketamine/valium cocktail into the cat's femoral vein. I knew how to do that! My hands didn't shake at all. Amy tapped on the cat's eyelid to ensure the palpebral reflex was absent, an indication that the amount of anesthesia sufficed. She then placed the cat on its chest, and stretched the neck up and forward into an arc.

She nodded toward some skinny rubber orange tubes and told me to choose the correct size for intubation. Holy cow, we'd never done that at Ralph or Andy's hospitals. I'd seen my bosses in Queens intubate a dog, but never a cat. They'd always used injectable anesthesia for cats, not gas. A cat's throat is tiny. I started to panic.

"I'll walk you through it," Amy reassured me.

I grasped the end of a slim tube with my right hand and peered into the cat's throat. I had no idea what I was looking for.

"Slide the tube down the trachea. Make sure you don't go into the esophagus."

That much I knew, as oxygen had to get to the lungs, not the stomach. I said a quick prayer and slid. Somehow it went into the right hole.

Barbara took over next, thank God, and hooked the cat's tube to the anesthesia machine. I had no idea how to work that thing.

I watched as Susan shaved the belly and vacuumed up the hair. Then she laid the cat on its back, tying each leg with a cord to a corner of the operating table. This looked like a horrific S & M scene.

"After you scrub up, Susan will help you put on your mask, gown, and gloves," Amy said.

I remembered seeing these accoutrements in movies, but not in any of the vet hospitals I'd worked in. I'd performed cat neuters and declaws with bare hands. I didn't remember the Joneses or Paco ever using a mask and gown, but they must have worn gloves at some point.

Amy led me to a specially designated sink, where she demonstrated how to scrub my hands with a nailbrush, using liquid soap from a dispenser. I had to turn the faucet handle on and off with my elbow so I wouldn't re-contaminate my hands. Susan held out a sterile paper towel for me to dry off. That was easy. My feathers fluffed, and I stood straighter. I felt professional and doctor-like.

After the scrub, I held my hands out like a zombie, careful not to touch anything. Susan helped me into a sterile paper gown and tied the straps behind me. She then put a mask over my face and tied those ends as well. When I was fully dolled-up, she pulled open the paper wrapper containing sterile surgical gloves. Amy pantomimed the correct way to grasp and pull on the gloves to avoid contamination.

Barbara scrubbed the cat's shaved belly first with iodine, then with pure alcohol. Amy told me to place the blue sterile drape over the cat's abdomen. Barbara handed me a scalpel. Amy said, "Cut a little hole in the middle of the drape, over the umbilicus." I slid the scalpel into the handle, as the doctor directed, willing my hands not to shake. I started with baby cuts, my motto being "better safe than sorry."

Amy corrected me, just as Elizabeth had. "Tiny cuts traumatize the skin. Make one firm continuous stroke."

"You can do it!" Barbara cheered, as she monitored the anesthesia. Susan smiled encouragingly as she handed me one surgical instrument after the other. I'm glad she knew what I needed; I didn't have a clue.

I forged ahead. Cats, unlike dogs, generally have very little abdominal fat, so it's supposed to be easy to find and isolate the ovaries. But I couldn't find either ovary. As loops of intestines and globs of fat bubbled up toward the incision, I fished around the innards with my metal spay hook. All I brought up were coils of intestine. No ovaries.

"Make your incision longer," Dr. Russell suggested. "It will be easier to find them that way."

I knew that vets prided themselves on how small an incision they made—an inch is considered good. Although I'd already exceeded that, I now tripled the length. I still couldn't find an ovary.

Amy glanced at her watch and gloved up to help me, as time is of the essence in surgery. The longer a cat stays under anesthesia, the more dangerous. Amy grabbed the spay hook from me, slid it down the near side of the abdominal wall, and immediately pulled out the first ovary. I fought a sinking, failing feeling. Amy didn't seem to notice or mind.

"Now you take over," she told me, "I'll walk you through it."

I had to clamp off the various arteries and veins with hemostats and then suture them tight, so when I finally cut through the tissue and released the hemostats, the cat wouldn't bleed to death. Amy stood by in case I needed more help.

After about thirty minutes later, I dumped the ovaries and uterus into a stainless-steel garbage bowl. Blotting the abdominal cavity with sterile gauze, I didn't see any seepage—so far.

Thank you, thank you, thank you God.

Almost over. I sewed the muscular layer with the purple stuff, which was slippery and harder to use than the catgut that I'd used in the other hospitals. When I questioned Amy about the difference, she told me that catgut (made from the intestines of various animals, not cat), cost a lot less than Vicryl, but caused a lot of inflammation to the tissue. Next I stitched up the subcutaneous layer, and finally, the skin, making the stitches as neat and even as I could. Still, the cat's abdomen looked like Frankenstein's face. I prayed my knots would hold.

Man oh man. Despite my winning the "Betty Crocker Homemaker of Tomorrow Award" in high school (they'd sure made a mistake with that one), sewing was not my forte. I wished I'd done better. In Home Economics, the worst thing that could happen was that a seam would open. Here, if I screwed up, the cat could die.

One final stitch, and I finished. I looked at the clock. One hour. A cat spay should take about ten minutes. My neck and back ached from hunching over so long. My nerves were shot. I didn't feel a shred of accomplishment, only relief.

Chapter 19

Two Hearts Opened

Later that month, Amy asked if I'd like to accompany her to the Bridgeport Animal Shelter. This was a municipal pound, a kill shelter: Dogs not adopted after two weeks were killed to make room for new arrivals. Amy wanted to get a couple of dogs to put up for adoption at the hospital. We'd each select one. Of course, I agreed!

Pet owners abandon dogs for many reasons: Cute puppies grow into unruly teenagers. Owners start a family and children replace the dogs. The responsibility of owning a pet sinks in—housebreaking, training, walks. Saddest of all is when owners dump older, faithful dogs—dogs they've had their whole lives—because they don't want to pay the medical bills that accrue with old age. These throw-aways pile up at shelters, as most people prefer to buy puppies from pet stores or breeders.

We dashed over to the pound during lunch break. As we approached, I heard dozens of dogs barking. When I stepped through the door, the stench of feces and urine assaulted me. I paused, allowing my eyes to adjust to the harshness of the fluorescent-lit, dank kennel. The sight of so many frantic dogs packed together, some three to a run, all vying for my attention, broke my heart. The dogs were soaking wet and kibble floated in their stainless-steel bowls. Apparently, the workers had recently cleaned the cages, accomplished by sticking hoses through the bars.

Amy told me to hurry, as we had to get back to work. This meant I had five minutes to decide which life I'd save. I raced down the long center aisle, glancing into each run. The dogs barked at me or stared at me—their eyes pleading. I had to avert my gaze. Only one dog. How could I choose?

I loved collies. I'd owned and devoured every single book of the *Lad: A Dog* series, Albert Payson Terhune's tribute to his collies. Terhune's collies were noble and kind, made of finer stuff than most people I'd known. I grew up watching *Lassie*, both the TV show and the movies. Lassie was a collie, his owner Timmy's best friend and protector. As a child, I'd longed for a best friend and protector. When I noticed a young Border Collie mix sitting quietly in the center of her cage, gazing at me with mournful eyes, my heart melted. The sign on her cage read something like Shada.

"This is the one," I announced to Dr. Russell.

When I walked the dog out of the shelter, she turned around to look at me. Her expression radiated joy and disbelief at her luck in escaping that prison. She jumped up and placed her two front paws delicately on my thighs and smiled in delighted amazement. She looked to be about six months old and thirty-five pounds, tall and slim. Her coat was long and wavy, all black except for two brown eyebrows, a patch of white on her chest and a little white snip at the end of her long, flowing tail. I named her Shadow.

Amy chose a golden retriever mix that she named Rainbow. We loaded the two dogs into the back of her car and returned to the hospital where we put them into the two cages she kept empty for adoptees.

That evening, before I left the office, Amy suggested I take Shadow home for the night. I couldn't bear the thought of her locked in that small metal cage overnight. So I agreed to take her to my tiny apartment.

I woke up in the morning to a big mess. Apparently, Shadow wasn't housebroken. Maybe that's how this sweet dog happened to be at the shelter on that late summer day. Whatever the case, the joy in her eyes made the cleanup worthwhile.

The next evening, as I prepared to leave work and to leave Shadow, her sad eyes followed my every move.

I never intended to keep her. I worked too many hours to own a dog, and my apartment was barely big enough for me. But I couldn't part with her.

She was as nice a dog as you can imagine, a perfect young lady. She *became* my shadow. When I left my apartment for just two minutes to take out the garbage, she threw herself into my open arms when I returned, whimpering in relief. In just a few days, I allowed my heart to open for the first time in my life. I let myself love Shadow the way she loved me. Our bond, mutual and unimaginably strong, felt like nothing I'd experienced before.

One day, as I stood in the park with Shadow, my heart overflowing with love and joy, I said right out loud, "I don't care, I really don't care, whether I find a husband or have children." I'd always expected to have a family. I'd read those adolescent romance novels along with the piles of dog and horse books that I'd checked out of the library each week. I'd longed for my Prince Charming, but I'd received only pain and betrayal from love interests over the course of my life. Lassie (and Shadow) would never betray me.

With the right combination of love, care, and nurturing, I would most likely have this amazing dog for the next fifteen years.

Outside of work, I devoted all my waking hours to Shadow's happiness. I rose before dawn each morning to drive the half hour to Compo Beach, where I'd unleash my baby. She'd race along the water's edge and chase seagulls and the waves for a full hour, while I kept a wary eye on her and watched the sunrise. Sometimes we'd go to Sherwood Island, a huge public beach and woods combination, open to dogs from October 1 to April 1. Dogs weren't allowed off leash, but early in the morning, or in bad weather, I'd risk a ticket.

One day, I received a letter from the New York Office of the State Board for Veterinary Medicine in Albany.

"Your written challenges along with a copy of your answer sheets were evaluated by the section chairpersons for the Small Animal and Bovine examinations. The score, which was originally reported to you on the Small Animal examination, remains unchanged. However, a passing score was achieved on the Bovine examination as a result of your challenge; therefore, you are now eligible for licensure in New York State."

I had studied two years for the New York boards. I'd been waiting for this letter for months. I had prayed to God for help for just this moment. I should have been thrilled, because I could now work in New York, but I wasn't. More than my own happiness, I wanted Shadow to be happy. She'd hate the city—she was a country dog.

On the days that the Russell Animal Hospital had no surgery, I'd race back to my apartment during lunch hour to walk Shadow. On surgery days, when I had to work through lunch, I hired dog walkers. But Shadow refused to walk with them. They told me she would lie in a catatonic state, barely raising an eyebrow when they arrived.

Besides Border Collie, Shadow must have had a little pointer or setter in her. I'd watch her stand stock-still if she spotted a squirrel. Without a peep, she'd focus on the poor little thing, lifting a front paw in a definite point. Then she was off and running. One day she caught one. The squirrel bit her on the nose and escaped. Whimpering, Shadow slunk back to me. I examined her closely for signs of injury but found none. Frantic, I asked my boss if squirrels carried rabies. They didn't, I learned to my relief.

Dogs and humans alike loved Shadow. She had the sweetest temperament and loved to play. Through her, I received and accepted invitations from other dog mommies to the theatre, concerts, lectures, or parties. Inevitably, though, I'd get an emergency call and have to cancel my plans. I hoped things would turn around, and I'd have some sort of social life. I still hoped to meet a guy and make some friends in my new hometown.

Shy and introverted by nature, I had to present myself throughout the day as an authority figure, projecting a confidence I didn't feel. Difficult cases and clients continued to challenge me. My highly educated Westport clients seemed to either be doctors themselves or have one in the family. In either case, they thought they knew more than me. And maybe they did.

I tried to keep up with the medical journals and to learn the newest drug protocols, but the information left me flat. I continued to dread surgery. I pushed myself at every turn, feeling the need to prove myself to exacting clients, and an exacting me.

When Thanksgiving rolled around, I finally had a day off, my first in three months. I couldn't wait to take the train to Manhattan to visit Grandma. I hadn't seen her since I'd moved to Westport a few months before, but it seemed an eternity.

Nostalgia swept over me as I headed toward Rockefeller Center where Grandma used to take me to the skating rink every Christmas. She'd lean over the guardrails and watch me practice my pirouettes and jumps. I'd feel pretty, like a ballerina, as I showed off my moves. Then we'd drink hot chocolate together at the outdoor cafe to warm up.

As I passed Saks Fifth Avenue, I remembered how each spring and fall Grandma would take me clothes shopping—either at Saks, Lord & Taylor's, or Altman's. She'd sit outside the dressing room on an upholstered chair and wait for me to show off the clothes. Grandma always complimented me on my figure and my looks, and sometimes, when I lifted my chin, turned a certain angle and squinted into the three-way mirror, I could almost imagine what she saw.

The doorman at the Carnegie House called up to Grandma, and so she stood waiting for me in her doorway. Taking my hand, she led me to the sofa. Her face glowed as she asked the inevitable question: "Where would you like to eat?"

"What about the deli?" I said.

Though I'm sure she wanted to take me to some fancy place for Thanksgiving, more than that, she wanted me to be happy. So she agreed.

We pulled on our coats and headed out the door to Wolf's Deli. Grandma hooked her elbow in mine, and we walked arm in arm across 57th Street. In Grandma's company, I felt so alive and present. Shadow and Connecticut seemed far away, like a half-forgotten dream.

The deli was empty. The hostess seated us by the window and handed us menus. I knew what I wanted, a cup of mushroom barley soup, so I didn't have to look. Grandma glanced at the menu and then ordered a pastrami sandwich.

"Is that all you want for Thanksgiving dinner? This is one of the best delis in the world—I bet you don't have anything like this in Connecticut!"

I didn't know; I never had time to eat out!

When the food arrived, Grandma said, "Take half of my sandwich; it's too much for me."

I looked longingly at the pastrami, but I declined, reminding Grandma that I didn't eat meat.

Grandma sighed and took two slices from a mountain of pastrami and put them on half a piece of rye bread. She changed the subject. "Don't you miss New York? You had so much fun when you worked here."

She sensed my ambivalence. In Westport, with work and Shadow filling my time, I'd forgotten there was more to life—until this very moment, enveloped in Grandma's love and breathing in the smells of deli pastrami.

"Now that you passed the New York boards, why don't you move back here where you belong? A single girl doesn't belong in the country."

I didn't answer but I sensed she was right. I was my best, true self here in New York.

She paid the bill, took my arm again, and, wordless, we walked back to the Carnegie House.

When the doorman held open the door, Grandma slipped him the remains of her leftover pastrami sandwich. I cringed. She always handed the doormen her doggie bag. I had no idea if they ate her left-overs or tossed them out, but they bowed in appreciation each time.

We returned to her couch, where Grandma put my feet in her lap and told me some *bubba meises* (a grandma's learned life lessons). Too soon, the antique gold-plated clock on the rosewood bureau struck 3:30. Time to catch the train. I had to be back in Westport to walk Shadow by 6 p.m.

Chapter 20

Just Like the Ashram

As I left the cocoon of Grandma's love and the familiarity of Manhattan, I had the eerie sensation of free-falling through a void. Gray freezing rain pelted the train as we pulled into the Westport station around 5 p.m. I made my way down the icy steps onto the slippery platform and located a trio of pay phones; thank God one of them worked. With frozen fingers, I called the taxi company whose number was glued on the phone booth. No one answered. Maybe Westport taxi drivers didn't work on Thanksgiving. I braced myself for the three-mile trek back to my apartment.

I trudged through desolate streets. Not a single store or restaurant was open. What a contrast from the energy of New York City.

When I reached my apartment and Shadow leapt into my arms, my world lit up again. The deserted, drizzly streets took on a magical glow as we took our evening walk. As I watched Shadow sniff the bushes, my heart swelled with love. There was nowhere else on earth I would rather be than with my dearest Shadow, the light in my life. We spent the remainder of the evening sitting side by side, watching TV. Now, New York City seemed the forgotten dream.

Still, after my chat with Grandma, I began to wonder whether I fit into life in Westport at all. Most of the women I met at the dog park, or through work, had husbands and children and lived in giant houses. They shopped and lunched, and maybe held part-time jobs, mostly as realtors, to keep busy. If the conversations weren't about pets, I had little to contribute. I'd rarely met people like these.

I'd never considered the size of one's house the measure of one's worth until I invited a new park friend, Hannelore, and her dog, Elle, to my apartment. She looked around with barely disguised pity. "I thought I had it bad," she said. After the divorce she'd downsized from a nine-thousand-square-foot mansion in Greenwich with a full staff, to a $2 million condo in Westport. I felt like Eve, realizing my nakedness for the first time.

I forced myself to attend a couple of singles functions, which I'd avoided like the plague my entire life. But I'd heard positive things about the Unitarian Church singles group. One evening, I gritted my teeth, got dressed up, and drove myself there for an event. I hoped that at least I'd meet other single women my age. No such luck. There was one man, whom everyone avoided, and the same middle-aged women I'd met at the park, most of whom were dumped by husbands for younger versions of themselves. Beyond dogs, we had little in common.

Baba taught the importance of keeping company with like-minded people, spiritual people. I decided to look for a Sai Baba center. I checked the Yellow Pages, inquired at the local new age bookstore, and scoured bulletin boards at health food stores. For weeks I came up empty-handed.

I finally remembered to pray. When I couldn't sleep at night, I'd fumble for the book of Baba's discourses that I kept on my night table. I'd randomly open to a page and inevitably see the perfect phrase for that moment—my reminder that God was near and listening. God had helped me to graduate, to pass the boards, and had led me to Westport. I had no doubt about that. Maybe my current challenge was how I viewed my life. I reminded myself, yet again, to have patience and faith, words I'd penned in neat block letters on loose-leaf paper and Scotch-taped to my bedroom wall.

The very next day, Jeff, a friend of a friend and a veterinarian, called to invite me to a collegial dinner. The first thing he noticed on entering my apartment was the picture of Sai Baba hanging on my living room wall.

"I know who that man is!" he said.

"Really?" I'd never met anyone in America who'd heard of Sai Baba.

"I did a house call for a woman yesterday who had his photos all over her house."

I knew this was no coincidence. The fact that God had orchestrated this dinner with Jeff electrified me. "Could you give me her name and number?"

True to his word, Jeff called me the next day and gave me his client's contact information. I called Suman immediately. She was president of the Sathya Sai Baba Center of Norwalk, the town right next to Westport! She invited me to their Sunday morning meeting, held at an Indian couple's house. I knew that centers were usually held in private homes because Sai Baba didn't permit money to be collected in His name—hence no funds for renting or buying space.

I counted down the days to Sunday when I drove to Norwalk and parked at the end of a double row of cars filling the long driveway. I made my way down a narrow concrete stairwell into the basement. Dozens of pairs of shoes neatly lined the floor of the windowless vestibule. I followed the strains of *bhajans* (Indian devotional songs) to an inner room and peeked in. Just like the ashram. The fragrance of incense filled the air. Fresh flowers decorated the altar. Men and women sat separate from each other, cross-legged on either side of the room in long columns.

Feeling conspicuous as the only white face in a sea of Indians, I took a seat in the last row of the women's section and gazed around in wonder. The scene transported me right back to Puttaparthi.

After forty-five minutes of singing, the group moved over crab-like to sit against the wall. I squeezed in between two sari-d women. Time for study circle. Lesson One for that day: "Problems and Worries are Only Passing Clouds." Oh boy, I needed to learn that one. Worry and anxiety took up a lot of real estate in my head. I fished around in my handbag and found a scrap of paper and pen to scribble down notes.

Lesson Two: "Praise and Blame all the Same." The world is a nest of crows; some caw in praise, some caw in derision. But people should be above the reach of praise and blame, Sai Baba said. In other words, don't be discouraged if some people blame you, and don't get puffed up when others praise you. We have to follow our Divine inner voice, the "still, small voice within," as it says in the Bible. Our conscience.

After final prayers, Suman came to greet me. We sat and talked for a while, and I admitted some of my fears and worries. She reminded me that thoughts were things, and I should think good thoughts if I wanted to reframe my life. She exuded what I longed for—spiritual wisdom. I left the meeting determined to put her words into action.

Chapter 21

A Friend and a Firing

The next day, an emergency call came in around 8 p.m., and I rushed over to the hospital. A pretty young woman stood outside the front door with a dying Chihuahua she'd just rescued from the Bridgeport Shelter. I ushered the woman and her dog into Room One. Colette, the client, chatted up a storm. We hit it off immediately. After I finished examining the dog, I told Colette to hang out in the waiting room while I brought Chiquita into the back, wrote up the record, and started treatment.

Colette and I had so much in common it was uncanny. A single Jewish lawyer, she'd just started her profession as a junior associate in a law firm. She was an animal lover dedicated to animal rescue. She was also a vegetarian. We even looked alike: five feet, seven inches tall, 125 pounds, long curly blonde hair, blue eyes, thin face, and athletic build. (Even her mother later said that I looked like the third daughter she didn't know she'd had.)

In short order, we became best friends. She owned three dogs: a three-legged Shepherd mix named Sherman that Colette had rescued from the Bridgeport Shelter; a severely arthritic Chocolate Lab, Tootsie Roll, a hand-me-down from her sister; and Chiquita, the almost-dead Chihuahua that I cured of Parvo.

Although also obsessed with her weight, Colette, unlike me, loved to cook. She made healthy, organic, low-calorie stuff, so I welcomed her almost-daily invitation—with Shadow of course—to dinner. My little girl was in doggie heaven chasing the squirrels and chipmunks on the acres of woods that surrounded Colette's cottage.

I'd sit at the rustic wooden kitchen table and watch Colette cut vegetables for our salad or tofu stir fry or pasta. Her perpetual cheerfulness fascinated me. How could someone always be so happy? Nothing seemed to get this Pollyanna down.

Her kitchen brimmed with food. I'd crack open her freezer and find my favorite Ben and Jerry's flavors: Chocolate Fudge Brownie, Chocolate Chip Cookie Dough, Chunky Monkey. I'd lift the lid off each pint to check them out. I'd want to sneak a spoonful, but they were all iced over. "Don't you ever eat these?"

"Not really. They're there just in case."

All types of goodies from organic chocolate chip cookies to organic blue corn chips (who knew corn came in blue?) filled her pantry. Colorful ceramic plates laden with organic fruits and vegetables sat on every counter. I noticed a huge bunch of bananas hanging from a special banana hook.

"Will you really eat all these bananas?"

"No!" She giggled. "I just like the way they look."

Her extravagance blew me away. I knew she earned the same as me, yet I bought two apples at a time and counted paper towels. "When they go bad, do you throw them out?"

She shot me a bright smile, "When they start to turn, I make banana bread. I love to bake."

Banana bread? Colette dieted and exercised just like me. "Do you eat the banana bread?"

"No, I freeze it, and if I don't have company for a while, they'll end up in the garbage."

One evening, after we finished dinner, Colette said, "Did you ever see a dog eat spaghetti?" I had not. Colette took the huge platter of leftover pasta from our dinner and called the dogs over. The four of them formed a perfect circle around her. She dangled a forkful of spaghetti above Tootsie Roll's head. Tuttie gobbled the strands from the bottom up. The others waited their turn and then sucked up the spaghetti, one after the other, in the exact same way. One forkful each and several circles round until the bowl emptied. Me, I would've reheated the spaghetti for three more meals.

Although we looked alike, there was a huge difference between us: Colette was an eternal optimist. Despite having a dysfunctional family, despite not having a boyfriend, despite living alone in an old rental, despite working ungodly hours for little money, despite all that we shared, she was happy. Each morning she'd wake up expecting the best—she told me so. I, on the other hand, waited for the other shoe to drop.

Driving down the dark country lane from Colette's happy house in Easton to my apartment one evening, my mind flashed back to seventh grade. I was standing in line for study hall feeling euphoric for absolutely no particular reason. A split second into that rare moment of bliss, I could hear my father's voice. "Life is serious. Be serious. If you don't work hard, you'll end up a failure, like your Aunt Carole." Dad worried about everything all the time, including his sister, whom he'd financially supported her whole life. I scanned my mind on that day in seventh grade, searching for a problem, any problem. My mind settled on an upcoming geometry test, and my soaring spirit crashed down.

I decided to reframe my perspective. I'd do my best to be positive, like Colette!

It worked for a week. Then Christmas rolled around.

Colette invited me to her big holiday party on Christmas Day, but I had to work, so I turned her down. Although we didn't see clients on Christmas, I'd still have to go to the hospital twice that day, as usual, for the weekend schedule to treat the animals.

The staff was abuzz the week leading up to the holidays. Apparently, Amy had given a Christmas bonus—an extra week's pay—to everyone. Except me. I asked Susan, the tech, why I didn't get a bonus. She told me that I'd have to work a full year to qualify. She looked smug. I'd put my heart and soul into my four months on the job so far. They could've at least given me a card.

On Christmas Day, when I walked from my car to the hospital entrance for afternoon rounds, I noticed a white envelope lying on the pavement in the parking lot. It contained three crisp, new $100 bills. I felt elated—then dejected. I knew it wasn't mine to keep.

The day after Christmas, I brought the envelope to work and asked if it belonged to anyone. It didn't.

Amy glanced up. "Keep it. It's probably drug money from the trailer park next door." (Yes, Westport had a trailer park.) She shrugged.

Maybe it wasn't a big deal to her, but it was exactly a week's take-home pay for me! My Christmas miracle.

For reasons unknown, Barbara, the tech, began watching me like a hawk at work. One morning after I'd examined a golden retriever with a hot spot, I excused myself from the client and hurried to the stairwell. I knew I'd prescribe prednisone and was pretty sure the dose was .25mg per pound, but I wanted to double-check in my little spiral notebook. I always wanted to be absolutely certain about dosages. I saw Barbara peer around the corner at me, but I didn't give it much thought as I rushed back to my waiting client.

That afternoon, Amy called me into her office. "What are you doing looking things up? You should know enough by now to get through a simple office call."

I wanted to disappear into the floor. "I just wanted to double check a dose," I mumbled. Honesty always seemed the best policy to me. Why conceal what I didn't know? But apparently insecurity was considered weakness here. Just like in the Fallek family.

I remembered seeing the film *The Way We Were* with my mother and sister during college break. As we walked back to the car, I bubbled with enthusiasm. "I loved the movie!"

"And I love Robert Redford," Mom had declared.

"Opposites attract," I said. "The fact that she was Jewish and he a Wasp had a lot to do with their mutual attraction."

"What the hell are you talking about?" Mom said.

"You are an absolute idiot," Debra chimed in. "That has nothing to do with it."

I slunk into the back seat while Mom and Debra took their places in the front, slamming the doors behind them. I braced myself.

"You think you know everything, don't you?" Mom snarled.

"I know something," I shrieked back, tears filling my eyes. "Why do you always condescend to me? I hate you!"

Mom looked at me with pure disgust. "If you have such a low opinion of us, how can you take our money for college? Don't you have any self-respect?"

Debra twisted around and glared at me. "You're a jerk; you don't know anything."

"You stay out of this! Mommy, tell her to stay out of this!" I started bawling. Tears were weakness and weakness was suicide, but I couldn't help myself.

"I'm not going to tell her any such thing," my mother said. "Look at you, just look at you. You can't take any criticism. Why don't you grow up? You're pathetic, always crying."

At work, the spying and tattling continued. When I'd enter the treatment room, Barbara and Susan would stop talking and smirk. If Amy was alone with one of them, they'd lower their voices as soon as they saw me. I'd seen this before, when they'd whispered about clients. I started to get a weird vibe.

When my six-month review came along, Amy called me into her office, her face stern. "Marcie, I'm not happy with your performance. What have you contributed to this practice?"

How much did I contribute? I worked seven days a week and was on call for emergencies every other weekend until 10 p.m.!

I'd admired Dr. Russell: She was an excellent vet, a real professional with high standards and expectations, and I had tried my best to live up to them.

She fired me.

I slunk out of her office with my tail between my legs.

Devastated, I picked up Shadow from my apartment and we headed to Colette's. She met me at the door with a hug. Then she made us dinner. "You're better off not being there anyway," she told me. She knew how diligent I'd been about my work.

When I got home, I stared at the words taped to my bedroom wall: patience and faith. Baba had said that troubles are only passing clouds. I hugged Shadow and prayed for the clouds to pass. As I cuddled with my baby on the living room floor, tears streaming down my face, somehow the gloom lifted and morphed into hope. Something better waited for me. I could feel it.

Chapter 22

"Kill the Kittens"

When the *American Veterinary Medical Journal* arrived in the mail, I went straight to the want ads. I found an opening for a veterinary associate in a town about forty-five minutes away and called for an interview.

Dr. Wentworth seemed like a kindly old country doctor, straight out of *All Creatures Great and Small*, the PBS TV show. Strangely enough, my firing turned out to be an asset, not a liability. As former head of the state ethics committee, Dr. Wentworth told me he'd seen his share of complaints against my former boss, and he offered me the job on the spot. He raised my salary and gave me a day off each and every week!

Working at his practice felt like a breath of fresh air. He trusted me with office calls and didn't mind if I looked things up or asked questions. I didn't have to hide my notes.

My first week also brought a surprise client: *The Man from U.N.C.L.E.* I'd had a crush on Robert Vaughn all during junior high. Although I was nervous, unlike with Paul Newman, I didn't call for the boss when this guy came in. Mr. Vaughn brought his new Bichon puppy in for an eye infection. Thank God, he didn't notice that I'd held the ophthalmoscope backward, shining the light into my eyes, and not into Peaches's.

I was as conscientious and meticulous as ever. A few weeks into my job, I received the results of a urine culture and sensitivity test I'd submitted for a miniature schnauzer. The results showed that the bacterial infection would respond to only one antibiotic. I couldn't find that drug in the office pharmacy, so I'd asked Dr. Wentworth if he'd order it.

"I'm not ordering any more antibiotics until we finish what we have." He turned and walked out of the room. What? The head of the ethics committee? I would've paid for it myself, but I'd just been fired from one job, and I didn't want to make waves. I gave the client something we had in stock. It wouldn't harm the dog at least, but it probably wouldn't work.

I made nice to everyone and tried not to step on anyone's toes. But the flirtatious young technician, Jennifer, gave me the cold shoulder.

A month into the job, Dr. Wentworth called me into his office. "Marcie, have a seat."

Oh no.

"I have a problem. I like you and think you are doing a fine job, but for whatever reason, Jennifer does not like you."

I felt sick to my stomach.

"I need harmony for the hospital to function smoothly. Jen has been here for years and fits in well with the practice. I'm sorry, but I'm going to have to let you go."

"When do I have to leave?" I managed to croak.

"Today is your last day. Feel free to use me as a reference. I wish you luck."

I grabbed my jacket, left the hospital, and stumbled to my car and back to the veterinary journal and classified ads.

I found an opening in a rich neighborhood about half an hour from my home. I'd heard that Jews weren't welcome in that neck of the woods, but I hoped no one at the practice would ask about my lineage, because I needed a job. I prayed for courage, collected myself, and called the place. The woman on the phone set up an interview for later that week.

I scoured my closet and dressed in the Waspiest clothing I could find: a khaki-colored, fitted, slitted skirt and a white, tailored, button-down blouse with a horse logo. I pulled on a designer brown jacket that I'd gotten almost new from Goodwill, then drove to the hospital. The place looked like a faux British stable.

I entered the waiting room. A make-up-less woman dressed more or less like me ushered me into an office and told me to have a seat. She was only a tech and clearly younger than me, but she made me nervous just the same.

She asked a few questions regarding my training and experience and jotted down some notes. When the tech finished writing, she looked up. "Dr. Martin will be right with you."

A lanky, middle-aged, clean-shaven man sporting a white lab coat and a serious expression entered the room. After unabashedly looking me up and down, he set the tone with the strangest comment.

"You do know we have a *certain type* of clientele here."

The type that doesn't want Jews?

This reminded me of the word "restricted" as used by country clubs and the like. Maybe he merely meant wealthy, famous people. But we had lots of those in Westport, and I'd never heard Russell or anyone else use that term.

The interview began. He presented two scenarios, the second so shocking that I forgot the first.

"A client calls up and makes an appointment to euthanize a litter of kittens. What do you do?" He eyed me coldly.

What kind of question is that? "I work with a rescue group," I said. "Everyone wants kittens."

"That's not the correct answer. If the client wants you to euthanize the kittens, that's your job."

Kill the kittens? Was he kidding?

End of interview.

What the hell was I doing in the veterinary world? I didn't fit in, at this practice or anywhere. As much as I'd struggled with vet school, I'd hoped that working in a practice would make it all worthwhile. I drove back to Westport, almost ready to give up fourteen years of my life. I hoped to God it wasn't too late to find another way to make a living.

Before the next batch of want ads came out in the new veterinary journal, I ran into Michael at the dog park. He was a fellow graduate from Bologna. I'd envied his situation. He worked for two kind partners in northern Fairfield County who were also excellent practitioners. It seemed that every time I'd met Michael, I'd be complaining about my job, while things sailed smoothly along for him. This time, it felt worse. I told him that I'd just been fired. Again.

"You're in luck," he told me. "I'm moving to Florida, and my employers will need to replace me."

His particular hospital never had to advertise. Their reputation was such that with word of mouth, the position filled immediately.

Michael may have called it luck, but I knew it was Divine intervention. Spiritual friends had told me that God waits until you're at the end of your rope to throw a lifeline—a test of faith thing. I needed that lifeline: I was sinking fast.

"I'll tell the guys tomorrow that you're looking for a job," Michael said.

He called me the next evening to say that his bosses awaited my call.

The interview with the partners, Alan and Mark, took place over lunch at a trendy restaurant near their hospital. The doctors met me at the door.

"You must be Marcie," Alan, a tall, bearded man with warm brown eyes said as he extended his hand.

"Hi there, so nice to meet you," said Mark, a short man with a strong New York accent and a genuine smile.

Their sincerity washed over me like a warm shower. The doctors hired me somewhere between the soup and the pasta.

Chapter 23

Like Brothers I Never Had

On my first day of work, Alan brought me coffee and offered to share his bagel. Mark greeted me with an effervescent, "Good morning!"

While I sipped my coffee, I asked the guys if there were any parks nearby to walk my dog. I'd brought Shadow with me, as time wouldn't permit me to run home at lunchtime to walk her.

When the doctors asked where she was, I replied that she was in my car, which I'd parked in the shade in the lot behind the hospital.

Mark looked concerned. "Bring her inside. You can put her in a run, in the boarders' section."

I appreciated the invitation but shuddered at the thought—all that barking and mayhem—she'd hate it. I explained to them that Shadow loved my car; it was her second home.

Alan bubbled with information. "There are lots of places to hike around here. My favorite is just down the hill—there are miles of trails in the woods." He told me that it had once been owned by the water company, but now that it was a state park, anyone could go there.

"There's another park about ten minutes from here," he said. "It's more of a playground for kids, but there's a swimming hole and trails toward the back."

Lunch break was from twelve to two, he told me, so I'd have plenty of time.

I couldn't be happier. Shadow would now have two-hour adventures each workday, which my bosses not only supported, but encouraged.

After coffee, Mark took me to my very own office, with a door and a desk and a space for my books; no need for cheat sheets on a stairwell. They gave me every single Wednesday off and, in the spirit of democracy, the three of us would alternate Sundays. I'd hit the jackpot with this job!

Not long after I was hired, Nancy, one of the receptionists, asked me for my birth date. I tensed. What did she want that for? Nancy giggled. "Don't worry, you'll see!"

Two weeks later, I saw.

There'd been much whispering that morning. "Don't leave at twelve for lunch," someone said. Another added, "It's Becky's birthday." They surprised her with a chocolate cake and full-throated birthday song, the likes of which I hadn't heard since I was probably five years old. Embarrassed by this show of affection, I stayed on the sidelines and only mouthed the words. No one left for lunch until we polished off the coffee and cake.

During slow times, I hung out with Nancy and her sister, both no-nonsense bespectacled women around my age who ran the front desk. Although they were the receptionists and I, the vet, we were peers in my eyes. We shared a love for animals and a dedication to work.

When time permitted, I'd trot downstairs to the lab where Martha, a chubby red-headed tech, taught me how to check for fecal and blood parasites and other things I hadn't learned in vet school or my prior jobs. During my tutorials, I tried hard to not space out during accounts of her trips to Orlando. Though Walt Disney World was not my thing, I preferred hearing about Mickey and Minnie any day to hearing gossip about clients and staff, which seemed to be a favorite pastime at other hospitals.

Each morning, Mark, Alan, and I would convene in the treatment area. First, we'd caffeinate ourselves, *kibitz*, and laugh. Then they'd quiz me about the previous night's *Jeopardy* questions. Both doctors loved *Jeopardy* and never missed a show. I couldn't care less about any game show (I'd always been a news junky), but these were my bosses, so having fun was practically an order. And it was fun. I didn't remember ever laughing so hard at 7 a.m. Even if I arrived exhausted and in a foul mood after another sleepless night, I'd soon be laughing. Mark and Alan felt like big brothers to me, not bosses.

Then we'd get down to business and discuss the hospitalized cases as if we were in a cabinet meeting. Many of the animals we examined together had been admitted the previous day. They'd been worked up with blood tests and X-rays. One by one, we'd pour over the intake and hospital notes and review lab results that arrived by fax at six each morning. After coming to a consensus, we'd move into radiology and mount the dog's or cat's X-ray on the viewing screen. Together, we'd plan a course of action. I felt validated, both as a person and as a veterinarian, to be considered part of the team.

Clients loved Mark. He schmoozed in the exam room and remembered the names of every client's kid and where they went to school. To me, his elfin ebullience seemed suspect. Besides Colette, no one I knew was so happy. But the staff assured me he was for real.

Alan didn't seem to need the limelight. Besides analyzing cases, he loved surgery and manual jobs. In addition to performing most of the operations, he took care of the plumbing and other repairs needed in the hospital. "Surgery, plumbing, carpentry, it's all the same," he'd say.

One day, Mark admitted a black Lab for observation. He hadn't figured out the dog's problem during the office visit, so he decided to keep the dog for the day. As the dog walked past, I noticed something odd. "Mark, isn't it weird how he's holding his tail to the side?" I asked.

"You know, you're right." He cocked his head at me, looking surprised and pleased. "You're very observant."

We examined the dog together. We discovered an anal gland abscess, which must have hurt so much that the dog kept his tail to one side.

Alan was a natural teacher who loved to test me. Late one morning, he completed a barium series on a vomiting corgi. With a barium series, a dog swallows the barium, an opaque contrast material, either via a syringe or via a stomach tube if the dog is anesthetized. A series of X-rays is then taken over pre-determined intervals, for example fifteen minutes, thirty minutes, and an hour, in order to follow the flow of the barium to find the source of trouble in the gastro-intestinal tract. Alan called me into radiology. He placed the first radiograph on the X-ray viewer and asked me what I saw.

"The stomach's filled with barium?" I said.

"Very good." Then he placed a second X-ray in the viewer. "What do you see now?"

"The same thing?"

"So why do you think it's the same?" he quizzed with a hint of a smile.

I hesitated. "There's something in the stomach blocking the dye?"

"Something's blocking the pylorus, so the contrast material can't empty into the duodenum. I gotta open him up."

Well, that made sense.

"What's all the raggedy white stuff under the vertebrae?" I added. Alan had taught me the importance of noting incidental findings on X-rays. ("Look at the whole radiograph," he'd say. He took the time and effort to answer my questions at every turn.)

"Very good! That's ventral spondylosis. There's too much stress put on the spine of these long-backed dogs. Bridging is the body's attempt to stabilize the back. Spinal arthritis can cause pain and eventually develop into paralysis. It's a good idea to bring this to the owner's attention."

I felt like an apprentice to a master, in clinical veterinary medicine.

Alan disappeared into surgery and came out an hour later holding up an apricot pit retrieved from the corgi. "A hell of an expensive pit," he said.

I could see he felt bad for the dog *and* the owner.

I recalled stories Joe and other colleagues had told me about certain hospitals. Some vets would admit a vomiting dog for an X-ray. If the X-ray was clear, the vet would place a quarter on the X-ray table under the dog, superimposing the coin onto the dog's stomach, so it looked like the dog had swallowed the quarter. The vet would then show the X-ray to the owner and tell them that the dog needed immediate surgery. Needless to say, this racked up a huge bill.

I'd seen one suspect ruse myself when shadowing a vet at a previous job. Someone brought in a dog with a marrow bone wedged in its jaw. I'd watched the vet lead the dog back into the treatment area and calmly slip the bone over the dog's teeth. The vet stuck the dog in a cage for the day and when the client returned, the vet presented him with a bill that included anesthesia, sawing off the bone, antibiotics, and hospitalization, among other charges.

What a relief to now work at a hospital where good medicine, and not money, ruled.

Most of the staff at this hospital had worked there since the partners took over the practice nearly twenty years earlier. This longevity was unheard of in the veterinary world. Given the long hours and low pay, most hospitals experienced a revolving door of technicians, receptionists, and associates. Alan joked that nobody in the office seemed to age, as everyone grew old at the same rate.

One day, Alan asked if I'd ever spayed a large dog. I told him I'd spayed a few cats, neglecting to mention that it had taken me an hour to do it.

"Would you like to try? I just admitted a five-year-old, ninety-pound Shepherd."

Spaying a big dog was a hundred times more difficult than a cat, and spaying was more challenging if a dog was large, old, or obese. This dog was all three. At least she wasn't in heat—that would have made it much worse. During heat, the tissue was friable. If you clamped it with a hemostat or tied it off with suture material, it could crumble.

I tried to feign enthusiasm as he led the dog into surgery for pre-op sedation. Alan asked me if I knew how to scrub and glove up. At least that much I knew. While I got ready, Alan knocked out the dog. "Yell if you need help. I'll be right here," he said, moving into the treatment area.

Patty, the tech, shaved and prepped Lucy, the Shepherd. I placed a sterile drape on the surgical site, took a deep breath and with slightly shaking hands, cut through the skin with the scalpel. So far so good. Then blood began to pool. I couldn't see my incision anymore. I stopped short.

"Blot up the blood with the gauze sponges," Patty instructed.

I had missed the linea alba—the fibrous tissue that connects the two halves of the abdominal wall—and cut through the adjacent subcutaneous layer and the muscle, causing the area to bleed. Gobs of fat popped out of the hole.

I fished around with my spay hook for a good ten minutes looking for an ovary, but all I caught were loops of intestine. (A typical Shepherd has about ten feet of small intestine.) I started to sweat.

"Help," I called out, hoping that Alan was nearby.

He rushed over and told me what Amy had said during my cat spay. "Healing is from side to side. If you can't find what you're looking for, lengthen the incision." I understood what he meant: Healing tissue forms perpendicular to the incision—the length of the incision doesn't affect the time it takes for a dog to heal. So, I should lengthen the cut.

"Be careful not to cut the bladder," Alan added.

I knew the bladder was somewhere down there, below the belly button. I extended the incision, but it didn't help. Ten more minutes of fishing, and I still couldn't find an ovary.

I called Alan for help once again. I didn't want to push my luck, but I also didn't want to keep the dog under anesthesia longer than necessary.

Alan rushed back, gloved up, and grabbed the spay hook from me. Despite his haste, he was patient as he demonstrated and explained. "I'll show you an easy way to find the ovary. You slide the hook along the body wall, facing caudally, then you sweep it up, like so, catching the broad ligament. *Voila!*" He clamped off one end of the ovary with a hemostat and stepped aside. "You take over," he said. "I'll stay here with you in case you need help."

Thank God he did. After I tied off the blood vessels and removed the hemostat, blood spurted out in waves from a pulsating artery onto my green surgical gown.

"Don't worry," Alan said. Unruffled, he tied off the artery and the gushing stopped.

The months passed, and I managed not to kill anything.

Chapter 24

Diagnostics and Detective Work

Every Sunday morning I'd meet Colette and friends and our pack of mutts at Huntington Park in Redding. Some altruistic artist had left her property to the town—eight hundred acres of woods, streams, reservoirs, and trails: doggie heaven. We'd see an occasional horseback rider or hiker, but beyond that, the park was ours. Shadow loved to chase animals, particularly deer, which scared the hell out of me. She'd disappear for ten, fifteen minutes but always came back, tongue lolling, deliciously exhausted. Despite my concerns, I couldn't deny her birthright. She was part Border Collie, so running was in her DNA.

In addition to her three-hour romp at Huntington on Sunday mornings, sometimes I took her for a late day jaunt to "the Barons," a dog park a few minutes from my apartment. They called it "the Barons" because it had been previously owned by a baron. Thirty-three acres of open space, with woods, fields, and trails. Another doggie paradise.

One evening, with the sun still bright and warm at 6 p.m., I spotted Colette's mother, Jane, and her two nasty Jack Russells at the Barons. Ignoring the dogs, Shadow ran straight to Jane, sat, and offered her paw, just like Lassie.

"Shadow's my favorite," Jane said, smiling, as she stroked my dog's head. Then Shadow noticed Portia, her husky/shepherd friend. All dogs loved Portia, but Portia loved Shadow best. They alternated between chasing and being chased. Shadow didn't care which—as long as she ran. After an hour, when the sun began to set, we headed home.

Although I was famished, Shadow's dinner came first, of course. A finicky eater, she'd turned up her nose at the Science Diet kibble our hospital had recommended. So, I tried Colette's method: I added some canned food and hot water to an expensive pet store kibble to make a sort of gravy, which she ate.

After dinner, Shadow was too pooped to jump on the couch, so I snuggled with her on the living room floor in front of the TV. By 10 p.m. I'd had enough of the news, so we moved to the bedroom. My twin mattress couldn't hold us both, so Shadow slept on a forest green L.L. Bean dog bed at the foot of my bed. Before going to sleep, I curled up with her on the floor for our nightly ritual. I cradled Shadow's upper body in my arms, lay my face on her chest, and asked, "Did Mommy ever tell you how much she loves you?" I didn't give her a chance to answer. "I love you more than anyone in the whole wide world! I love you more than my life. I love you more than life itself." I kissed her warm soft eyelids, first one then the other, over and over with baby kisses, until she exhaled with contentment and fell asleep. I kissed the tip of her cold wet nose and climbed into my bed.

The next day, while I dressed for our morning walk, Shadow looked up at the skylight and sighed. I knew that sigh. She longed for the outdoors. I vowed to find her a house with a yard someday.

Things were going well at work, and I had no reason to fear being fired a third time. I did well in office calls; I was a good diagnostician. I took thorough histories, paid close attention to detail, and dismissed nothing the owners told me. I cared. The clients seemed to like me, and so did the staff.

As much as possible, I'd sit or crouch on the floor with a dog rather than tie them to the scary metal table with a noose. I stroked the cats on the table, reassuring them, rather than restraining them. I'd seen vets and vet techs at other hospitals manhandle animals into submission and it had cut straight through my heart. I treated the dog or cat with the respect they deserved, as kindred souls. I considered them sentient beings, as worthy of love and compassion as humans. I knew they felt my love.

I never rushed an appointment and examined every square inch of the dog or cat. I preferred chronic cases, especially ears and skin, to emergencies.

Treating ears proved perfect for my OCD: I'd meticulously clean out the ears, making sure to get out the last bit of debris. Other vets usually just dispensed Panalog, a generic antibiotic. Leaving nothing to chance, I'd culture the discharge each time, in order to choose the most appropriate antibiotic.

Lots of vets disliked dermatology because curing skin problems seemed an insurmountable task. Month after month, year after year, the dogs and cats would return with ever-worsening skin disease. To cover most of the bases, vets usually prescribed prednisone along with antibiotics and anti-fungals—the kitchen-sink approach, I called it. But I enjoyed the detective work necessary to figure out the underlying cause. I'd scrape, culture, biopsy, try them on a hypoallergenic diet, use an Elizabethan (cone) collar, add some natural supplement I'd read about, do whatever it took, with as little drugs as possible in order to avoid side-effects. Generally, my patients seemed to improve.

When office calls ran smoothly, I felt on top of the world. One morning, I entered exam room Number 2, feeling very pleased as the Post-it on the record had my name on it. I entered, not to a smiling owner, but to an irate return client, his face red with anger. Looking straight at me, he snarled that his dog had an ear infection that I'd obviously overlooked two weeks earlier during our office visit.

I started to shake. It hadn't been there two weeks before, and I told him so!

"Now I have to pay for another visit because of you!"

When he left, I ran to the back in tears. Alan looked up in surprise. "What's the matter?"

I explained.

"Don't take things personally," he said, returning to a husky's cruciate surgery. "I once had a client who screamed constantly at my staff. It was so bad that his wife would call after every visit to apologize for his behavior. During one of his phone rants, the line suddenly went dead. I had no idea what happened. I forgot about it. I found out later that the client had a heart attack during the call and died. How people act is a reflection of themselves, not of you. Remember that."

My wise and supportive boss. I adored him.

Once, when I'd expressed a touch of jealousy over his big house, pool, and boat, he'd flashed me a wry smile. "The more things you own, the more things own you."

Still, I wanted a house with a yard. Mostly for Shadow.

In December, Colette found me a six-hundred-square-foot house rental in Fairfield that allowed pets: two rooms and a galley kitchen for $1000 a month. In Fairfield County, this was a steal.

The kitchen was a Depression-era original. I figured I could paint over the rotting wood and Con-Tact paper the drawers, like I'd done in college. The long narrow bedroom could accommodate a single bed, a small dresser, and a bookcase. The living room had a picture window, which didn't open, but plenty of sun streamed in. An old, screened-in porch stood at the far end of the house, so I figured I could leave the back door open for air. The layout didn't make sense to me. But it sat on a nice piece of property. The two-hundred-square-foot backyard where Shadow could hang out was totally fenced in and bordered by bushes.

But no bathtub. That could've been the deal breaker. I had tried washing Shadow in a shower, which turned out to be impossible. I told the landlord that I'd sign the lease on the condition he put in a tub.

With an extra month's pet deposit, the landlord conceded. The apartment would be ready in three months. I signed the lease. I couldn't wait to show Shadow our new home.

Chapter 25

A Crash Splits the Air

One picture-perfect autumn day, Alan invited me to join him on rounds at his pet stores, followed by lunch. I knew he co-owned two pet stores, but I'd never seen them. How could a girl say no to her boss's invitation for lunch?

"I'd love to!"

I felt horrible that Shadow would miss her midday walk, but I stifled the feeling. Before we left, I ran out to the car to check on her. She was fast asleep. I promised myself I'd make it up to her later.

I hated when pet stores sold puppies because I knew where they came from: puppy mills, industrial breeding facilities usually located in the Midwest. Proprietors of these abominations packed dogs in stacks of filthy cages, churning out litters season after season. The mothers and puppies never touched paw to ground, never played with toys or enjoyed any human contact. When the bitches were too old to breed, they were killed.

I'd often examined these pups at their initial puppy visits. They tended to be riddled with problems. Many of them had been on continuous rounds of antibiotics for chronic respiratory infections, diarrhea, or skin disease. Some owners complained that their pups had trouble walking. When I'd questioned my bosses, they'd told me the problem was temporary, caused by the pups' confinement to the metal grates of their cages. After a couple of weeks of walking on firm surfaces, the legs would straighten out, they said.

As Alan drove the half hour to his pet store, my mind wandered from puppy mills to pet stores to dog rescue and to my work with New Leash On Life, the animal rescue group Colette and I had started after I was fired from my Westport job. Colette and I and about fifteen other women gathered for our meetings on the first Saturday of each month at Bloodroot Restaurant in Bridgeport, a feminist vegetarian restaurant/bookstore that probably hadn't changed since the sixties. We'd order food from the hand-written chalkboard and carry our tiny, overpriced organic meals on a tray to our family-style table. We'd eat off of unmatched pottery and drink herbal tea from the chipped ceramic mugs we'd select from the old wooden breakfront.

After dinner we'd squeeze into the cluttered meeting room. We perched on any available space—the floor, the arms and seats of broken-down sofas and armchairs, or on rickety wooden chairs. Amidst the chaos, we plotted and planned. Our goal was to help the dogs and cats at the Bridgeport Shelter, many of which traced their origins from pet stores and puppy mills. Our motto—*Save a life: adopt, don't shop.*

On the Saturdays that we didn't meet, we would volunteer at the Bridgeport Shelter, each contributing what we could. Colette, president and resident attorney, navigated the significant liability obstacles. Lisa, the handiest, fenced in an area so that the dogs could socialize and exercise. Linda, the dog groomer, bathed, clipped, and shaved the dogs, transforming them from walking disasters to clean, adoptable lookers. I took care of the dogs' medical needs. We took turns walking the dogs and scrubbing down their cages. Our work culminated in a yearly summer fundraiser, a dog show, emceed by Colette and attended by hundreds. Every dime we raised went to the care and feeding of the dogs at the shelter.

Alan held the door open for me as we headed into his store. I couldn't help myself; I had to ask: "Alan, how can you support puppy mills?"

"My puppies come from private breeders, not puppy mills," he insisted, no further comments forthcoming.

I had my doubts but kept quiet.

I followed Alan into the back office where he introduced me to his part-ner at the pet store, Chris, a Ken-doll look-alike. Alan told me to make myself at home and relax while he examined and vaccinated the caged puppies, but when he and Chris left the room, I spotted some American Kennel Club documentation on the desk and went over to investigate. I checked carefully for any puppy-mill affiliation. Sure enough, the "breeders" were all located in the Midwest.

Half an hour later, Alan returned. "Are you hungry?" he said.

I nodded.

"One more pet store, then lunch."

I made myself let the puppy-mill thing go, and we laughed non-stop over my vegetable bean curd soup and his three-course special.

Back at the hospital, I rushed to my car and peeked in the window. Shadow was still asleep and apparently hadn't even noticed I'd been gone.

After work, Shadow and I headed home. The route took us past the Barons. Shadow stared at me, her eyes bright with expectation. I hesitated. The sun was beginning to set, which concerned me, but I felt guilty that I'd made her miss her midday walk.

I'd never risked taking Shadow there in the dark, because I feared she'd run off. But Shadow was such an obedient dog, the envy of all the dog owners at the park. Running free, off leash, she'd turn on a dime to come when I called. "Why can't you be more like Shadow?" I'd heard more than one owner chide their disobedient dog.

I turned to her. "OK, OK. We'll do one short loop. Just once around!"

We got out of the car and walked toward the woods in our normal clockwise direction. Half-way around the park, I made out the form of a deer in the growing dusk, at the clearing on top of the hill. I'd never, ever seen a deer at the Barons. I froze in horror—North Compo, the adjacent road, would be filled with rush-hour traffic.

I looked back at Shadow, but she was gone. And so was the deer.

I screamed, "Shadow, Shadow!"

Suddenly a loud crash split the air. The impact jarred me to the bones. I ran toward the road, sure that a car had hit the deer.

Then I saw a black heap lying by the side of the road. I dashed over.

My baby, my world, lay at my feet.

I stood in shock over her perfect, unmarked, beautiful body, which lay motionless on the asphalt. A stream of blood trickled from her mouth.

My screams echoed in the darkness.

I bent down, and with tremendous effort, slung Shadow's body around my shoulders in a kind of fireman's hold. I struggled under her weight as I headed to my car. Only then did it occur to me that I could've driven my car to her body. But I could never leave her alone like that. I laid my little girl in the back seat, her bright red blood soaking the powder blue upholstery.

I drove home, shell-shocked. Should I take her body up the stairs? Or leave her in my car until I could put her in the freezer the next day at work? Once a week, a cremation service made the rounds, collecting bodies from the freezers.

I left her in the car and managed to call Colette, my voice cracking. "Shadow is dead. A car hit her at the park."

"Stay where you are. I'll be there in twenty minutes."

I paced up and down outside my apartment. Colette came as promised. She took my car keys and drove us to the all-night emergency hospital in Norwalk.

I turned away as the techs carried Shadow's body into the building.

"Why don't you sleep over at my house tonight?" Colette said. "You shouldn't be alone."

I accepted Colette's offer and made up the futon in her spare bedroom. I closed the door, turned on the TV, and lay on the bed, fully clothed. News of a 6.9 earthquake in San Francisco flooded the airwaves. Images of the wreckage in that beautiful city mirrored the devastation and grief in my heart.

The following day was a Wednesday, my day off, but I couldn't bear to be alone. I called work, told them what happened, and asked if I could come in. Everyone at the hospital gave their condolences. I trailed the staff as they worked. After work, I returned to my empty apartment.

I couldn't bear to look at anything Shadow, so I threw it all away. Her bowls, her bed, her toys, her leashes. In the days and weeks that followed, I'd occasionally find a tuft of black on the floor and weep as I pressed her fur to my lips.

I drowned my grief in my work, where no one at the hospital mentioned Shadow again.

Chapter 26

A New Business

When Thanksgiving rolled around, Mark invited me over to celebrate with his family. He'd told me that I reminded him of his eldest daughter—"idealistic and smart"—and said he looked forward to introducing us. I'd never had a boss who understood the essence of my nature. Touched and flattered, I wanted to accept Mark's invitation, but I called Grandma first to ask if she'd mind.

"You're lucky to have such a boss," she said, giving her blessings.

On Thanksgiving Day, I sat at the kitchen table with Cynthia, Mark's wife, as she made last-minute preparations. We talked life and reminisced about the old country—New York. I felt right at home, as comfortable as if I were with Grandma. I looked around for the family's Standard Poodle. "Where's Gigi?" I asked Mark when he joined us.

"I didn't want her underfoot, so I left her in a run at the hospital."

Gigi was such a docile, well-behaved dog. Wasn't she family?

Later, around the dining room table, I chattered on non-stop and ate way too much. I had planned to leave by 9 p.m. but surprised myself by staying until 11.

As soon as I drove out of their driveway, I burst into tears. Where had this come from? I'd just had a great time. Then it hit me: I couldn't recall one meal where the Fallek family had sat around and talked as if we liked each other. Grandma had told me many times, "I've never heard a kind word spoken in your house. I've never seen anything like it." I hated the screaming and fighting, but it was all I'd ever known.

With Mark's family, I'd felt like I was in an old-fashioned movie, like *Little Women*, or a part of a TV show, like *The Waltons*. Once, when I was around eight, I'd slept over at a friend's house. The father had died, and the two sisters and mother acted like best friends. It had felt so strange. I kept waiting for something bad to happen, but it never did.

The day after Thanksgiving, I shook off the loneliness and continued reinventing my colleagues as my surrogate family.

Over the weeks, after work, with no reason to go home, nobody waiting for me, I threw myself into back-to-back ballet classes, returning to my apartment just in time to collapse into bed. Life felt empty and meaningless without a dog. I asked my broken heart, was it really such a sin if I bought a collie? But deep in my soul, I knew I couldn't, I just couldn't. I couldn't live with myself if I didn't practice what I preached. I had to rescue a dog in Shadow's honor. So I combed all the shelters within a hundred and fifty-mile radius from home, driving to a different shelter each day. On workdays, I checked out nearby pounds. On my days off, I traveled for hours.

In the meantime, I found something to fill the void. One day, Judy, a lapsed vet tech and ex-breeder of Bull Mastiffs, brought a pregnant bitch into the hospital for a C-section. Judy and I hit it off and decided on the spot to start a part-time house-call business together: she the tech and I the vet. Multi-pet households naturally preferred vets to come to their house, rather than having to *schlep* the whole pack to the hospital. Judy told me she knew lots of people with lots of dogs and puppies, which all needed yearly vaccine boosters. I checked with the bosses and they didn't mind. Judy and I set a date to discuss our new venture.

When the day arrived, I drove to Judy's home in Wallingford. A dozen mild-mannered, hundred-pound-plus dogs wandered the property. She had outdoor runs and a fenced-in yard for most of the animals, with a few lucky dogs as house pets. Her place was nothing like the puppy mills that I'd read about or seen on TV.

Judy admitted as we walked the property that she'd generally lost money on breeding. She did it because she loved the breed. Bull Mastiffs give birth by C-sections, a costly procedure. Food and medicines for these huge dogs ran up correspondingly huge bills. "What are those hills at the edge of the lot?" I asked her.

"Dog poop."

She piled the feces along the fence line and then planted grass seeds on top. Half a ton of dogs produced a corresponding amount of poo.

Judy put on a pot of coffee and we sat at the kitchen table to strategize. First, we set about creating a price list. We agreed to follow the hospital's fees, with a 10 percent multi-pet discount, and then added a charge for the house-call. We would split our fee down the middle.

We already had a first client: her niece's Rottweiler had a litter of twelve, which needed first puppy shots. I did the math. I would bring home almost a week's salary from that one house-call!

At the appointed time, her niece, Sarah, welcomed us inside and took us to the living room, which was bursting at the seams with Rottweilers. I proudly took my new $500 otoscope and $200 stethoscope from my back-pack. I opened a red plastic lunchbox that my mother had given me, which I'd filled with icepacks and vaccines, and set to work. I examined and vaccinated the puppies one by one, recording the information carefully into a treatment record. I handwrote an individual health certificate for each puppy, detailing their date of birth and my physical exam findings, then pasted the sticker from the vaccine vial next to their name. One hour later, after declining a cup of coffee, I left with a pocketbook stuffed with cash.

More important than the easy money was the feeling of appreciation. Sarah hadn't stopped thanking me from the moment I'd entered her home.

Word spread and our house-call practice grew. I made professional business cards and even got some solo vet work. Slowly, I was learning to trust my knowledge and listen to my inner voice.

During my off time, I continued to search for a dog. One day, I visited the North Shore Animal League on Long Island in New York, the largest no-kill shelter in the world. If I couldn't find love there, I couldn't find it anywhere.

Although I arrived an hour before they opened, dozens of people had already queued up. When the attendant opened the door, I pushed past the crowd in the puppy section. Puppies weren't my thing. It could be difficult to judge a dog's character at such a young age, and I wanted to know what I was getting. I made my way to the adult dogs. I strode up and down the corridor, pausing at every pen to look deep into the eyes of each face—the windows to the soul. I sought an intelligence shining from the eyes and a soul-to-soul connection.

All day long, I watched people come and go. It astonished me how quickly they chose their pets. Most wanted a puppy. Many wanted a purebred; some kind of status symbol, I guess. Others wanted a dog that resembled the one they'd lost. The rare saintly person, like Colette, chose a special-needs dog—deaf, blind, or paralyzed.

At the end of the day I was losing hope as I had already seen more than a hundred dogs. During one last turn past the runs, a scrawny heap of black matted hair raised its head. The dog hadn't looked up on my first two rounds. But this time, our eyes locked.

I signaled to a young female attendant.

"That's the one I want, the 'spaniel mix' (which looked to me like a Dobie) with the plaque labeled 'Jingles.' It says, 'check with staff.' Is she taken?"

The girl eyed me closely. "She's not a 'looker' but she's our favorite. We all love her! She's smart and full of personality. We wanted to make sure she got a special home."

She took "Jingles" out of the run and handed me the lead.

The dog had no tail.

I'd been obsessed with tails since I was little. Long flowing manes and tails on horses, fluffy brown and white tails on collies, wagging tails, proud tails. I used to tie a scarf around my waist and pretend I had a tail. Without a tail, a dog seemed barely a dog!

Conflicted and distraught, I went to the pay phone and called my mother.

"Your best friend, Colette, has a dog with three legs. What the hell does it matter if it has a tail?"

I knew she was right. I shoved my obsession aside and renamed the dog Annie. My little orphan Annie.

They placed Annie in a holding pen, while I filled out the paperwork. She stood up on her hind legs, watching me intently as I disappeared into the office.

She was too weak to jump into my car, so I lay her down on the passenger side next to me. But she had other ideas. She crawled toward me, cramming her twenty-two-pound skeletal frame into my lap. I idly stroked her, resentment building that this dog was alive while my Shadow was dead. I pushed these terrible thoughts away and focused on the road.

After our dinner of eggs and pasta, all I had in the apartment, Annie settled in at the foot of my bed, where she slept peacefully the whole night, while I lay awake, fearful she would disturb my sleep. At the crack of dawn, I leashed her and walked her down the narrow stairwell to the street. As soon as she hit the sidewalk, watery diarrhea poured out of her. As a veterinarian, I knew the self-control it took for her to not mess the house or wake me for a walk during the night. Her sweet thoughtfulness touched me.

I brought her to work the next day, not trusting her alone at home with colitis. Plus, I wanted to show her off, the fruit of my weeks of searching.

Alan was the first to see her, and with his usual bluntness said, "Where did you get that mutt from, the basement? So many beautiful dogs in the world and five weeks of looking: this is what you brought home?"

Chapter 27

Get Used to It Now

One day, a client dropped off a young cat for a routine dental cleaning. I examined the cat, listened to the heart—normal—and determined he was healthy. I sedated him with an IV pre-anesthetic.

The cat stopped breathing.

Horrified, I yelled to Alan. "The cat just died!"

Alan ran in, tapped the eye, and listened to the heart. He put an oxygen mask on the cat's muzzle and pumped on his chest. No change. He grabbed a syringe and injected something into the heart. The cat was still dead.

Alan turned to me and shrugged. "These things happen. You'd better call the owner and tell her."

Call the owner? "Please, can't you call her?" I begged.

"The hardest thing you'll ever have to do as a vet is to tell the owner that their pet has died. You better get used to it, and you may as well start now." He gave me a few pointers of what to say and left.

My heart pounding, I dialed the owner's number. My voice quivered. "Mrs. Anderson, I'm so sorry to tell you that Moses passed away."

"What? Aaaaaiiiiiii!" she screamed into my ear.

I rattled off the talking points that Alan gave me. "We're not sure why he died, but when an apparently healthy cat dies under anesthesia, there's usually an underlying problem." I tried to sound professional, but inside, I was dying myself.

I wasn't sure that she heard me above her wailing, but I persisted and asked for permission to perform a necropsy, which is an autopsy for animals. Through choked sobs, she agreed.

Alan came back into surgery when he'd heard I'd finished the call. Under his watchful eye, and with his direction, I opened the cat's chest and pulled out the heart. "Now slice right through the ventricle," Alan told me. "I bet you'll find it's severely hypertrophic (thickened). Nine times out of ten, when a young, healthy cat dies suddenly, for no apparent reason, it's due to hypertrophic cardiomyopathy."

I sliced through the heart. The ventricle walls were so thick there was barely any room for blood in there. Poor kitty. Any amount of anesthesia would probably have been fatal. While I was still sad the animal had died, I was also relieved because this wasn't my fault. I called Mrs. Anderson with the news. (Good news for me, not so much for her.)

The following week, Alan admitted a dog that had been hit by a car. "How would you like to try a leg amputation?"

Not at all. "Sure," I told him, bolstered by his faith in me.

Alan intubated the boxer mix, hooking him up to anesthesia. The techs shaved and prepped him, while I scrubbed up.

Dear Alan stood right by me, guiding me every step of the way. Cut. Tie. Cut. Tie. It was backbreaking work dissecting the tissue and tying off the many vessels. It took me over an hour to separate the leg from the body.

"Good job."

Though Alan complimented me, I felt not one iota of satisfaction. In fact, I wanted to puke as I eyed the leg.

On the heels of the leg amputation, Alan offered me the opportunity to behead a cat after we put it to sleep, which is the only acceptable method to check for rabies. I politely declined. I didn't even want to watch.

After he finished, Alan called me in to show me his handiwork. I nearly fainted when I saw the cat's head lying in a box of dry ice, ready to be sent to the lab in Hartford, where they'd check its brain for the virus.

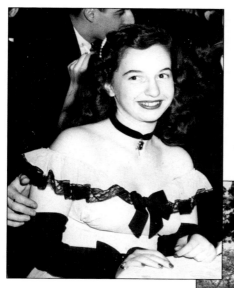

Mom, Marilyn Schreiber Fallek,
who was Miss West End Avenue
before marriage

Dad, Jerome Fallek,
before marriage

Marcie at twelve years old,
on vacation in Paris with
sister Debra and Mom

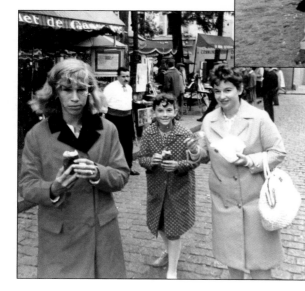

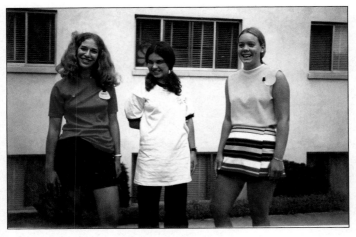

First day at Emory University with roommate Debbie and another friend

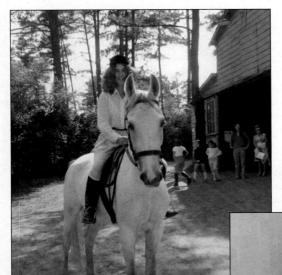

Riding a Lipizzaner in a horse show while at Emory University

In her apartment in Bologna, scraping the flesh off of cow and horse bones to prepare for anatomy class

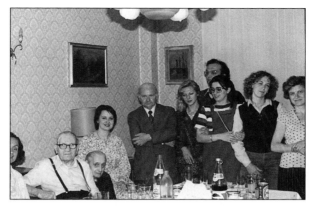

Outside Bologna, among Italians seeking spiritual guidance
from a psychic medium

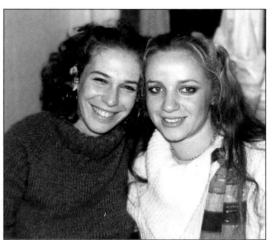

With friend Gy in Bologna apartment

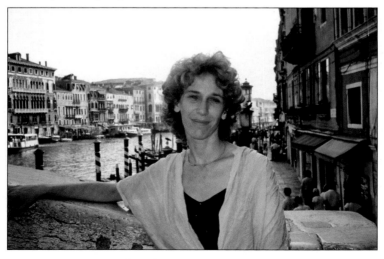

Visiting Venice on a rare day off

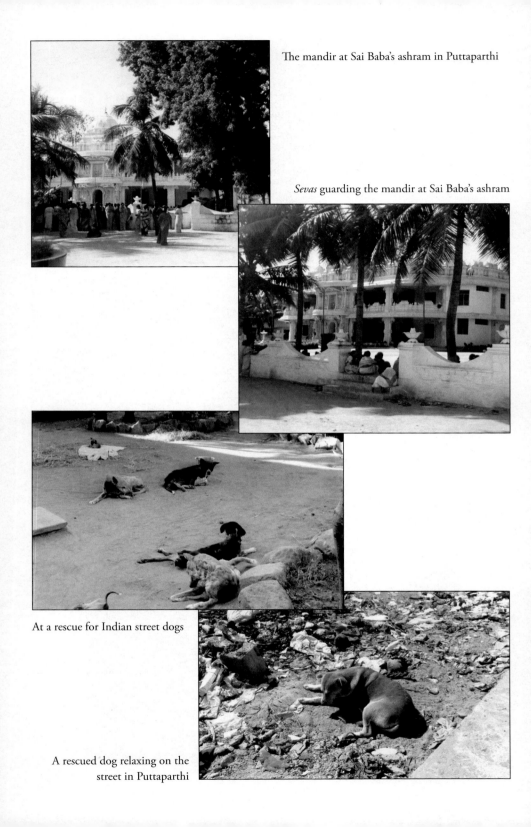

The mandir at Sai Baba's ashram in Puttaparthi

Sevas guarding the mandir at Sai Baba's ashram

At a rescue for Indian street dogs

A rescued dog relaxing on the
street in Puttaparthi

Rear entrance to the ashram depicts symbols of the world's five major religions

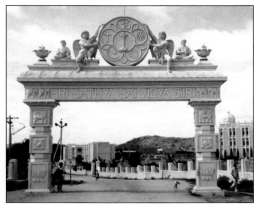

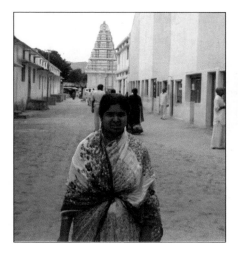

At ashram, a fifteen-year-old girl who, devotees say, was resurrected three days after her death

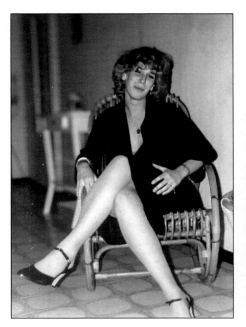

Dressed for the "meeting" with Professor Morro

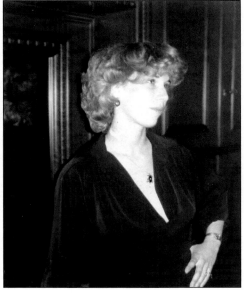

Steeling herself to meet with the lecherous professor

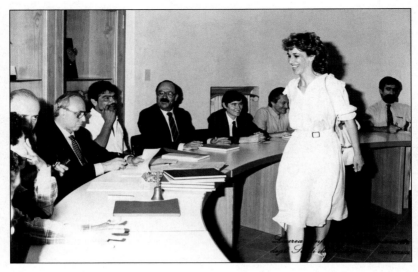

In her clearance-sale Dior dress after presenting her thesis on graduation day

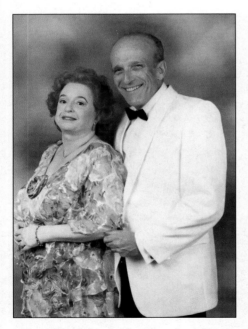

Mom and Dad shortly after Marcie's graduation from vet school

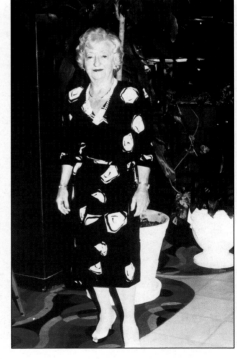

Grandma Betty Schreiber vacationing in the "Borscht Belt" in the Catskills, New York

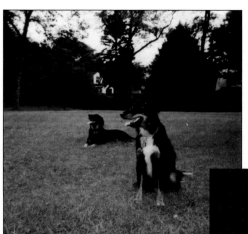

Shadow, in the foreground, at the Barons

Annie, at friend Colette Griffin's cottage

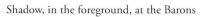

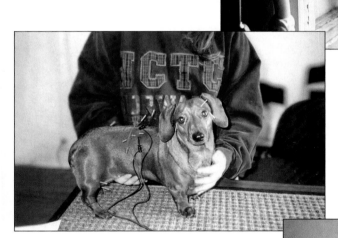

Acupuncturing a dachshund with a herniated disc

Acupuncturing a client's dog,
Sierra, to help relieve her anxiety

Rocco, the boxer puppy who was headed for euthanasia due to "untreatable" demodectic mange, post-acupuncture at his happy forever home

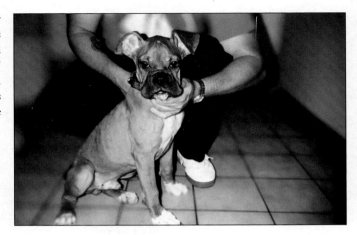

Marcie's Rottweiler mix, Annie, after one of many ACL surgeries

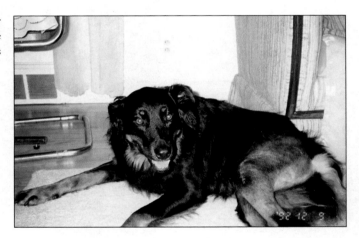

A homeopathic consultation for a Golden Retriever with Irritable Bowel Disease

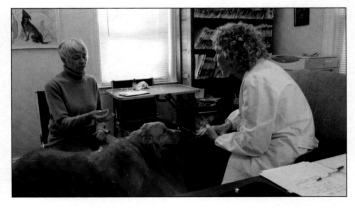

The partners eventually understood that I hated surgery. So we settled into a routine. One partner and I would do office calls in the morning, while the other partner performed surgery. In the afternoon, a partner and I would do office calls again while the morning's surgeon took the afternoon off.

Though I managed to avoid surgery, there was another procedure I hated but couldn't avoid: euthanasia. I hated everything about it. I didn't feel right taking a life, even though I knew at times it could be the kindest option. Plus, dead bodies gave me the creeps.

For me, the absolute worst was when the owners wanted to be present. Like the day the Davis family brought in their miniature poodle, Charlie Bear, to put to sleep. Like many poodles, Charlie Bear had lived a long life. He looked every bit of his nineteen years. He was in end-stage kidney failure, blind, deaf, and cachectic (wasted).

Mrs. Davis cradled Charlie Bear in her arms, while Mr. Davis spread someone's shirt on the cold metal table. The two kids bawled non-stop.

Becky gently took the dog from Mrs. Davis and placed him on the shirt. She held off the vein so I could inject the euthanasia solution into the cephalic vein. Now all four Davises started crying. As the family hovered over Charlie Bear, hysterical with grief, my shaking-hand syndrome reared its ugly head.

"It's Charlie Bear's time," I said, making a desperate attempt to still my hand. No good. I missed the vein. Charlie Bear shrieked. The pentobarbital had leaked into the subcutaneous tissue, which I knew burned like hell. Missing the vein also meant the vein was blown—meaning I couldn't try that vein again.

The whole family stopped their crying, stared at the dog and then at me. My blood ran cold. With a tight, apologetic half-smile, half-grimace, I mumbled something to the effect that Charlie Bear was severely dehydrated, so his veins were tiny and difficult to hit.

I gestured to Becky to move to the dog's other front leg. We took our positions once again. All four Davises resumed their crying. Sweat poured down the small of my back, and my hand shook even worse. I took aim and injected. Charlie Bear shrieked again. *Shit!* The family now glared at me.

My mind raced through my options. He had two rear leg veins, but they would be even harder to hit than the front ones. I'd had the unfortunate experience of using up all four legs in the past and didn't want a repeat. I excused myself and ran into the back. Thankfully, Mark was free and said he'd take over. He went into the exam room with the clients. I'm not sure what he did or how he did it, but a few minutes later he returned with the body. He didn't look upset with me at all.

Unfortunately, they didn't let me off the hook for future euthanasia.

One day, after a *successful* euthanasia, just as the owners' tears abated, the dead dog sat up, like in a horror movie. Everyone shrieked, especially me. I'd seen involuntary twitching and spasms of the muscles after death, but nothing like this. I thought the dog was going to jump off the stainless-steel table. Instead, he fell flat down again.

Chapter 28

A Punch in the Gut

I never thought I'd love again the way I'd loved Shadow, but Annie, that little ragamuffin, grew on me. She was intelligent, confident, and loving. On December 1, she and I moved into what should have been Shadow's house.

Following months of drug and food trials, Annie's diarrhea resolved, and she transformed from an emaciated Dobie mix into an eighty-five-pound Rottweiler-Australian-Shepherd, a real character, grounded and sure of herself. More human than dog, she knew exactly what she wanted. When we walked around town, alone or with company, she'd stop at each intersection and look around. I could see the cogs turning in her brain: she was deciding which way to go. I always let her choose. With time, even Alan admitted that this former heap of matted fur was a fabulous dog.

One day, a fellow dog mom from the Barons told me about another local dog park, Lake Mohegan. I couldn't wait to bring Annie. On my next day off, we made the twenty-minute drive. As we approached, Annie stood in her usual position, rear legs in the back, front legs on the center console, staring out the windshield, tongue lolling in a big open-mouthed smile. Once out of the car, she raised her head, sniffed the air, and rushed deep in the brush, a woman on a mission. Two minutes later she returned with a tennis ball in her mouth and then led the way on the winding dirt path to the lake.

Once we reached the water, Annie looked around and dropped the ball in the sand. With the tennis ball firmly between her paws, she dug a hole with ball and paws. She took the now sandy ball back in her mouth, shook it vigorously—as she would if breaking the neck of a small rodent—and ran into the lake. She dunked the ball several times in the water then came ashore. I watched in astonishment as she repeated the sequence two or three more times. When she finished, she turned to me with a big grin. For the life of me, I couldn't figure out what she had done. But clearly, she knew, and was extremely pleased with herself.

Annie could swim. I knew that for sure, because I'd send her to retrieve objects even the Golden Retrievers and Labs couldn't find in the lake. All I had to do was point. Like a submarine, sure and certain, she'd head laser-focused for the tennis ball or stick. But when she got hot, instead of swimming like Shadow, she'd wade like an old lady. She'd walk into the lake up to her chest and swish her *tush* in the water, cooling it off, beaming up at me the whole time.

And boy, could that girl eat! Although I didn't eat meat, Annie had to. Dogs need meat to maintain good health. Even though we sold prescription diets at the hospital, I refused to feed her this stuff. I researched the ingredients and found it to consist of animal waste-products condemned for human consumption, artificial colorings and flavorings and lots of words I couldn't pronounce. Instead, I bought her the best organic, preferably free-range meat I could find. She'd inhale it, along with a mixture of organic grains and veggies, mixed with extra virgin olive oil and a vitamin/mineral supplement that I made up each day. I'd mix it together in the first food-processor I ever owned. Annie always stopped midway through the meal—about five seconds—to shoot me a wide grin.

Soon after Annie and I settled into the house on Smith Street, Alan brought a beautiful ten-week-old Seal Point Himalayan kitten to the hospital from his pet store. I couldn't take my eyes off of her.

In Bologna I'd fallen in love with Persian cats. (Himalayans are Persians with Siamese coloring.) Persians suited me perfectly. They had a calm and loving disposition, the opposite of your clichéd aloof, hyper-active feline. In Italy, I'd adopted a blue/gray Persian I named Tabu. Originally owned by a breeder, Tabu hadn't produced any kittens, so the owner wanted to get rid of her. She'd returned to the United States with me after graduation, but when I moved to Connecticut, I left her with my parents in Lido. I knew she'd be happier in the big house than in my cramped, windowless apartment.

Alan looked me in the eye. "I have to put her to sleep."

"Why?" I gritted my teeth, mentally condemning pet stores.

"Her brother tested positive for feline AIDS, so it's not ethical for us to sell her, or even give her away."

"I'll take her!" I knew she might have AIDS, but I didn't care. AIDS isn't necessarily fatal in cats. They can stay asymptomatic for years.

"I hoped you'd say that!"

I forgave Alan and cuddled my new blue-eyed piece of fluff. I named my new kitten Shanti, which means peace in Hindu, which was, after all, what I sought.

Life seemed to be settling into place. A new house, a job I loved, and my little family of three.

Then one evening, my mother called with bad news: Grandma had lung cancer, and Mom was bringing her home to Lido to die.

What?

I felt as if someone had punched me in the gut. Now I understood why Grandma had gagged and coughed during our recent phone calls. The choking spells had frightened her. I had reassured her that it was nothing, but in my heart of hearts, I sensed it was something bad. Still, I was in denial. I needed her to live forever.

I rushed to Lido that Wednesday, my day off. Mom hadn't told Grandma she had cancer.

(Grandma had always said that if she ever got it, she wouldn't want to know.) Grandma wondered why Mom had rushed her to Lido with a suitcase full of stuff.

When Grandma was out of earshot, Mom said she'd known about the cancer for over a year. I was crushed. How could Mom keep this from me?! I wasn't a child anymore to protect from "secrets." I'd taken the time with my grandmother for granted. I could never get that time back. Now, every moment with Grandma would be even more precious. During my visit, we ate dinner together downstairs in the kitchen. The following Wednesday, I made another three-hour drive, and, when I arrived, Grandma was lying in my bed and couldn't get up.

I returned each Wednesday.

During my sixth and final visit, Grandma sat in a wheelchair by the window. She hadn't eaten in days and could barely breathe, an oxygen tube keeping her alive. Tears welled up as she looked deep into my eyes and gasped her final words to me: "I know how you feel. And I feel the same way."

Our unspoken "I love yous" unleashed my tears. We sat in silence listening to the humming of her oxygen machine until I had to leave.

We had a very small funeral. I cried alone. My family barely spoke of her again.

I threw myself into my work, same as when Shadow died. But I'd wake up in the middle of the night howling with grief. I hadn't realized how much I depended on my Grandma. While I lived in Italy, years would pass without seeing her, but I was OK with that. I knew she loved me. Merely knowing she was alive and breathing somewhere on this earth had sufficed.

Depression began to settle over me like a heavy winter cloak. Thank God for Annie. Each day after work I'd lay myself on Annie's eighty-five-pound frame and soak up the love. I could count on Annie 100 percent, just like Grandma. I called her my Rock of Gibraltar.

But one day, out of nowhere, Annie's knee seemed off. (Dogs have two knees and two elbows, just like us.) She had a hard time walking so I brought her into the treatment room for Alan to check out.

"I think Annie ruptured her cruciate ligament," I told him.

"Why do you think that?"

"By the way she holds her leg."

"Let me have a look," he said. Alan bent down and felt her knee. "Doesn't look like anything, but let's put her under and take an X-ray after lunch."

We studied the radiograph together. I didn't know what I was looking at, but Alan said it was non-remarkable and probably just a sprain. "Put her on NSAIDS (non-steroidal anti-inflammatory drugs) for a week, and she'll be fine," he said.

No way, I thought. Although I'd studied conventional medicine and dealt with pharmaceuticals for a living, personally, I avoided drugs. I knew from experience that drugs had side effects—seizures, paralysis, liver failure, kidney failure—which I was careful to spell out to my clients. I may have dispensed them, but they were not an option for my baby.

Besides, I didn't believe Alan's diagnosis. I knew this was more than a sprain. I just knew it. With the blessing of my bosses, I took Annie to Dr. Bill McCarthy, the best veterinary orthopedic surgeon in Connecticut, for a second opinion. I'd referred lots of animals to him over the years and loved this big teddy-bear of a man, even if he did hunt with his pure-bred Labradors.

Dr. McCarthy fit us in the next day. He greeted Annie by name, just like I did with my clients. He had me walk her up and down the corridor while he watched. Then he kneeled down and carefully felt both knees. Afterward, we reviewed the X-rays I'd brought with me. He repeated Alan's verdict: soft tissue injury—Annie was fine. He told me to rest her and give her NSAIDS.

I disagreed but was relieved that the specialist thought she was fine. I rested her—no long walks, no trips to the park—but refused to give her the drugs.

I called Mom for her advice.

"Remember that newspaper article I cut out for you?" she said.

I did remember. Mom had sent me a *New York Times* article about a veterinary acupuncturist. I'd glanced at the article and stashed it away with other stuff in one of my huge to-do piles. She knew my proclivity for natural medicine. After all, I'd sporadically seen acupuncturists and naturopaths for my insomnia over the years, which she'd paid for.

Though a veterinary acupuncturist in 1990 was virtually unheard of, Dr. Russell and I had referred a few dogs to one in Greenwich. Not one of them had improved under his care. Still, a veterinary acupuncturist could be an alternative to drugs and surgery. Maybe it was time to give it another try. After I hung up with Mom, I searched for, and found, the article.

I figured if the *Times* wrote about him, he had to be good.

Chapter 29

A Curious Cause

As I read the article, a calm descended on me. This veterinarian was spoken of as a healer. To me, a healer was touched by the Divine, like Jesus. I knew a bit about acupuncture. The notion of healing with energy resonated a heck of a lot more than prescribing pharmaceuticals. I felt a paradigm shift, and I called the acupuncturist's office to set up an appointment.

That Wednesday, I drove fifty-five minutes north on country highways, buzzing with anticipation. I entered a no-frills, cramped waiting room, filled with animals and their people. It appeared that Annie and I had a long wait, so I filled the time eavesdropping on conversations. I heard miraculous stories from grateful owners: Paralyzed dogs that now walked. Dogs in need of hip replacements that now ran pain-free. Chronically ill, formally drug-dependent animals now drug-free and thriving. I felt like I was in Lourdes! What a difference from the chatter in our own waiting room, where tense and fearful clients commiserated over the sad details and fate of their pets.

When Annie's name was called, a receptionist ushered us into an exam room. I crouched on the mat with Annie, eager to meet this famous healer. A few minutes later, Dr. Paul Hoffman entered. With long hair, beard, and jeans, he looked more like a hippy activist than a typical veterinarian. My kind of guy.

He looked at me, then my dog. "What's the matter with Annie?"

"I'm pretty sure she ruptured her right anterior cruciate ligament," I told him. "I'm also a vet," I added, self-conscious, not wanting to appear a show-off, but feeling I had to explain my medical knowledge.

The doctor raised his eyebrows.

"I don't want to give her painkillers, or have surgery," I explained. I felt weird saying that as one vet to another, but given his specialty, I figured he'd get it.

The doctor asked me to have Annie stand and hold her still. He knelt down and ran his hand along her spine, pressing gently. Then he stood behind her, and placed one hand on either knee.

"Yup, the right knee is thicker than the left. Now walk her around the room." He watched carefully. "See how she slightly favors that right leg, and toe touches when she stands still? I think she has a tear."

I knew it! How extraordinary, that he could diagnose a ligament rupture with only his hands and eyes, versus manipulating the knee under anesthesia, like we conventional vets insisted.

He put Annie's X-ray in the viewer. After studying it for a bit, he turned to me. "Did Annie have a Lyme vaccine recently?"

What did that have to do with anything? I scanned my memory. "Yeah, I think she had her booster a couple of months ago." I followed protocol like everyone else.

The doctor pursed his lips. He said that, in his opinion, the Lyme vaccine was not only ineffective, but also dangerous. He told me it could have been the cause of Annie's knee issues.

What?

I'd been taught that ACLs, or cruciate tears, were caused by acute injuries. In fact, ACLs are known as "football knees" in human medicine. This didn't add up, though, as Annie never ran. She strolled. Part Rottweiler, she was built like a tank, not an athlete.

Dr. Hoffman explained that ACL tears can also be due to a chronic degeneration of the joint, caused by auto-immune disease; in other words, an out-of-whack immune system in which the body attacks its own tissues.

"The Lyme vaccine can trigger auto-immune disease," he said.

I knew he was confiding in me, professional to professional. He scribbled down the name and number of the top veterinary immunologist at Cornell University veterinary school. "Give him a call when you get home," he said. "He'll be happy to talk to you."

Vaccines could cause ACL tears? I found this hard to wrap my head around. I'd always been skeptical of drugs, but never doubted the safety and efficacy of vaccines. In fact, I spent most of my workdays and my now thriving house-call business administering them!

I'd been taught that the cause of autoimmune disease was *idiopathic*— no one knew what caused it. Various theories were proposed, such as stress, genetic predisposition, and medications, but no one really knew. I did remember a vaccine insert listing a few side effects of vaccines, including a warning that the vaccine could cause autoimmune hemolytic anemia (that's when the body destroys its own red blood cells), but that was extremely rare, according to the manufacturer's warning.

The notion that vaccines could be dangerous shocked me, but I believed this vet. He had nothing to gain by sharing this information. On the contrary, it could anger the veterinary board, as well as trigger the ire of his colleagues. After all, vaccines were a huge source of income for vets.

Could I have contributed to Annie's lameness?

Dr. Hoffman went to a narrow, overstuffed cupboard in the corner of the room and took out a small cardboard box with Chinese writing on it. He told me to keep Annie on her feet. I watched, fascinated, as he inserted razor-thin gold acupuncture needles along her spine and in her knees. She didn't flinch. In fact, she visibly relaxed. After he'd placed about twelve needles in her, he told me to have Annie lie down. She settled comfortably and he attached wires from a portable contraption to the needles on her knees. "Keep her still," he said. "I'll be back in twenty minutes."

I sat on the floor with Annie and stroked her, relaxing into the strange peacefulness of the place. Not a single bark or howl broke the calm.

Dr. Hoffman re-entered the room with a smile. As he removed the needles, I asked how acupuncture worked. There were two theories, he said. According to the Chinese, energy runs in meridians throughout the body. Disease occurs when there is a blockage of energy. Acupuncture restores the normal flow, bringing the body back to homeostasis, or health. The Western scientific explanation, he said, was that the needles release neurotransmitters and hormones such as serotonin and endorphins, strengthening the immune system and initiating a healing response.

"Which theory do you believe?" I asked.

He hesitated. "Both." He told me that certain acupuncture treatments consist of placing only one needle in a very specific point for that particular individual.

How intriguing! Each subsequent Wednesday at the acupuncturist's office, I overheard more success stories in the ever-packed waiting room. The clients raved about this miracle-worker. They seemed to place him at the right hand of God.

After each session, I'd ruminate and daydream on the drive home. Despite five years of practice, I still didn't fit in the veterinary world. I hated surgery, I didn't trust drugs, and after a half-hour phone conversation with the vet at Cornell, I began to question vaccines.

I wondered if my time at my job was limited as well. Alan and Mark didn't want another partner, and I'd already outlasted their previous associates by a couple of years. Not a single one of those vets had made it past two years. The partings had been mutual, I'd been told, as the guys (yes, the associate vets had all been men) had left to start their own practices. I assumed that Alan and Mark also preferred paying novice vets a correspondingly lower salary. I'd gotten a steady 6 percent increase every year, and now made almost $40,000.

Could there be hope for me elsewhere?

Dr. Hoffman used acupuncture, Chinese herbs, and other natural supplements in his practice. During my Wednesday sessions, I plied him with questions, which he did his best to answer while shuttling between exam rooms. Six weeks into Annie's treatment, he surprised me. "How would you like to work for me?"

Would I!

"But first you must take the IVAS course and become certified in acupuncture." He told me that a new session of the International Veterinary Acupuncture Society would be offered in the fall in Atlanta. The course consisted of six, five-day modules given over the year.

Since meeting this vet, I'd fantasized about carving out a similar path, but hadn't a clue how to begin. Now, it seemed, providence had laid it out for me, in a fashion almost too good to be true.

My body buzzed with excitement. I'd never for one moment felt as enthusiastic about my profession as I did now.

Chapter 30

A New Path Appears

I took stock of my professional life and began to envision a new path. I'd always felt like a square peg trying to fit into a round hole. Each month I had to force myself to tear off the plastic cover of the AVMA journal. (It put me to sleep.) I was reluctant to celebrate a successful outcome of some drug therapy, as I was wary of the yet unseen side effects. Yes, prednisone seemed to help a lot of conditions, but even the so-called experts admitted that long-term administration of pred devastated the body. It caused muscle-wasting, suppressed the immune system (predisposing the animal to infections), and caused endocrine diseases like diabetes and Cushing's disease and many other disorders. And I still felt no sense of accomplishment after completing a surgery—only relief that I had gotten through it without killing the animal.

I cringed when vets discussed euthanasia in front of their animal patients. When I tried to shush them, they laughed at me. I shuddered for hospitalized animals when vets performed necropsies of other pets right in front of them. When vets joked and laughed as they killed and cut, I was horrified. I felt that the animals understood, if not the words, at least the tone. I could see it in their eyes.

One morning, Alan arrived late. He apologized and said that his dachshund, Maggie, had just been killed by a car in front of his house.

I stared at him. "You don't seem very upset."

"Why is everyone telling me that?" he exploded. "I cried when it happened. What more do you want?"

I'd rarely met a vet in America who loved animals. Italian vet students had been different. Veterinarians there didn't make much money (bank tellers made a heck of a lot more). Many of the vets I'd met in Connecticut and New York seemed indifferent, at best. Others even appeared to actively dislike animals. (Of course, that's not what they projected to the clientele.)

Love and concern for animals had been my motivation for attending vet school. I wanted to heal with love, like the lady in *The Three Lives of Thomasina*. But love of animals, except among the techs and receptionists, didn't seem to be the driver in any hospital I'd worked in.

I respected my bosses as professionals, but questioned the detached way they regarded even their own dogs. When Mark stuck Gigi in a run to get her out from underfoot at home, she would languish there, until a tech reminded him to take her home.

I hated the runs, those three-by-six-foot concrete cubicles out back where the partners stashed boarders as well as large, post-surgical dogs. Granted, they were better than cages. At other hospitals, even overpriced, fancy ones like the ones on Park Avenue in New York, they shoved big animals into small cages, so in comparison, our facility could be considered palatial. We had a separate cat room, too, an amenity that I'd never seen in the veterinary world.

Elsewhere, when pet owners lovingly handed over beds and toys to hospital staff at admission, the animals never saw them—most hospitals stored them in cabinets so they wouldn't have to wash them before returning them to the clients. At least we gave the stuff to the pets.

But the boarders still looked miserable. They barked and howled or lay depressed and inert. Mark understood their plight. He referred to them as the "general inmate population."

Not a single veterinarian I'd met in the States understood why I didn't eat meat. "I don't eat my patients," I'd joke in response to their tiresome queries, as we sat around conference banquet tables—they with their steaks and me with my plate of vegetables. Other than a title, we seemed to have nothing in common.

For reasons I didn't understand at first, my bosses kept a "hospital dog" in a run out back. Nellie was a sixty-five-pound tri-colored coonhound whose sole purpose was to donate blood to anemic hospitalized dogs. This had been required exactly three times in the four years I'd worked there. Her pitiful, resigned expression broke my heart. Couldn't we keep frozen blood, or refer the anemic dog to a bigger hospital for a transfusion? Couldn't we use one of the staffs' or partners' dogs if a transfusion was needed? Apparently not.

There'd been much chatter recently among the techs. The partners had added two more coonhounds out back. Every so often, a harried man with a foreign accent and a truck would collect the two hounds. Sometimes the dogs came back. Sometimes they didn't. Then we'd get another pair. No one knew what was going on.

One day, I overheard Mark and Alan discussing the coonhounds: they were being used for experiments at a local human hospital. Coonhounds' and beagles' placid natures make them perfect candidates for vivisection— operating on them for experimental purpose—so they are often bred for this. The reason for the replacements, I learned, was that sometimes the dogs died during the process. I didn't know if it was the anesthesia or the experiment itself that killed them.

I confronted Alan and told him that I thought it was disgraceful that we participated in this atrocity. I'd always been against animal experimentation, but I'd only read about it. These animals' lots in life seemed worse to me than the starving dogs in India. At least the Indian dogs were free and living with their pack. They had hope.

Alan told me that experimenting on dogs helped save human lives. "Animal experimentation saves children," he said. "Children with cancer," he repeated in a sanctimonious tone.

I told Alan that I loved my dog as much as he loved his son.

The practice continued.

Many vets, I imagine, viewed their profession as a profitable business venture. Several vets had told me they'd wanted to be medical doctors but couldn't face the many years of internship and residency, as well as the astronomical cost of liability insurance. But Dr. Hoffman seemed to have a different motivation. When he treated Annie, he talked about the importance of "intention" in acupuncture. I understood this to mean that love and a selfless desire to help the animal would create the best results.

This had always been my intention.

Could intention really determine a certain outcome? If you put a needle in the correct point, shouldn't it work no matter what you were thinking? Were needles even necessary?

I'd seen hands-on healings. I'd even experienced one. In Italy, I'd gone to a ninety-two-year-old energy healer. I described the migraine-like headaches I'd get from lack of sleep. He stood behind my chair, placing his hands outside of my temples. I could feel the energy flow from his hands right into my head. Then and there the headaches disappeared, and they never reoccurred! So, the concept wasn't new.

But from a veterinarian? I thrilled at the thought.

In my experience, vets eschewed alternatives, particularly anything that seemed metaphysical. Maybe they'd entered vet school like that, or maybe their training produced this way of thinking. Either way, most didn't—or couldn't—think outside of the box.

But I believed that we, living creatures—humans and animals—were more than just a heap of organs and enzymatic processes, more than the sum of our parts. Call it soul, or whatever word resonates. I believed there was something greater at work in this universe and maybe this was my chance to tap into it. I believed that all healing ultimately comes from God. I'd witnessed this again and again. Weren't we, all of us, instruments of God? And so, Divine?

In one fell swoop, as I envisioned a new path with Dr. Hoffman, the spiritual me merged with the professional me.

At the eighth acupuncture session, Annie still showed no sign of improvement. Healing was a process, Dr. Hoffman had said at the outset. Give it eight weeks. Some dogs, he'd told me, didn't respond at all.

"Should we give up?" I said.

Dr. Hoffman frowned. "At this point I think you should consider surgery." Though my heart fell, I'd suspected this was coming.

He told me to biopsy Annie's synovial membrane, which would determine if the ligament rupture stemmed from a trauma or was *immune-mediated*. In other words, from a vaccine.

As I was about to leave, Dr. Hoffman turned to me. "Come here as often as you can to observe," he said.

I couldn't wait to attend the IVAS course, but first I'd need permission from my bosses. Because my job had taken precedence over everything in my life, I'd never considered asking for an extra day off, not even when Grandma was dying. I was immensely grateful for all that my bosses had done for me, and I didn't want to take advantage of their generosity. But I'd need six free weekends in order to attend the certification course, and Alan and Mark were protective of their weekends. Over the past four years, the partners had allowed me only two Saturdays off per year—the ones included in my two-week vacation.

I stood at a crossroads. I didn't want to miss the course and lose the opportunity to work with Dr. Hoffman, but I had a sinking feeling that the four Saturdays could pose a problem. Still, I had to take the risk. Even if it meant losing my job.

I caught Mark between patients. He agreed to meet with me and Alan after morning appointments.

"You guys know I've been taking Annie to an acupuncturist for the past couple of months." I willed my voice to remain calm, ignoring the semi-deafness caused by my tightening Eustachian tube. "That vet told me about a certification course. In acupuncture for veterinarians. I'd, um, I'd like to take it."

"Sounds interesting," Alan muttered, shuffling through a large stack of papers.

I forced myself to keep talking. "The thing is the course has six modules. Every couple of months I'd need Tuesday through Sunday off." (I'd need an extra day for the flight.)

Alan shot to attention, stared at me, and then glanced at Mark. "That means you need six Saturdays off?"

I nodded.

They looked grave. "We need to discuss this," Alan said. "We'll get back to you in a day or two."

I was dispensable; I knew that. But God had helped me through other obstacles. I hoped He wouldn't let me down now.

The next day Mark gave me the OK.

Chapter 31

Ten Bucks an Hour

The following Wednesday as I drove to Dr. Hoffman's, I felt like I was floating on a cloud. Finally, I'd met a veterinarian who was "cut out of the same pasta" as me, as they'd say in Italy: a kindred spirit.

The receptionist smiled in recognition and ushered me into the treatment area where Paul sat on a stool eating lunch. He glanced up and continued shoving pieces of celery into a small container of hummus, and then shoveling it into his mouth. This was a first. I hadn't seen another vet eat hummus for lunch. I wondered if he was a vegetarian.

I asked how he was. He mumbled a few syllables through a mouthful of food. I took the hint and shut up. Maybe eating was a meditation for him.

After polishing off the last bite, he looked me straight in the eye. "Don't speak when you come into the exam room with me, don't ask any questions, and don't talk to the client." With that, he left the room.

Huh? What was going on? He'd invited me here to learn. How was I supposed to learn if I couldn't ask questions?

I followed him, robot-like, into Room One.

"How's Buddy doing?" Paul gushed.

"Great! He's starting to use his back legs, thanks to you, doctor." Mrs. Levine beamed.

The miniature dachshund, like so many other doxies, apparently had disk disease.

"Excellent. As we discussed, in a couple of months he should be as good as new."

They chattered on while I plastered myself against the door, trying to make myself invisible.

Paul caught my eye and pointed his chin toward the dog. I crept into position—left hand under dog's neck and right hand under the belly. I stared at a gold-framed diploma on the far wall.

I shifted my gaze as often as I dared, to watch. Paul inserted gold-colored acupuncture needles along the dog's spine and into the rear legs, much as he'd done with Annie. He hooked the needles to the electrical machine and then ordered me to keep the dog still. With that he left the room.

Blood pounding in my ears, I turned toward the owner with a tight-lipped smile. She smiled back. We took turns smiling at each other for the next twenty minutes.

Finally, the door swung open and Paul entered. I unfroze my smile and lowered my eyes. He checked the dog and removed the needles.

He faced the woman. "Next Wednesday, right?"

"Yes. Thank you, doctor. I'm so grateful for all you've done."

"You're most welcome." He flashed her a bright smile.

She left with a wave.

The doctor turned from her and pushed through the connecting door into the second exam room. The swinging door whacked me in the face as I tried to follow.

What had changed? Dr. Hoffman had been so nice to me when I was a client. Why was he now so cold? I equated being holistic with being kind and compassionate—not only to animals but also to people.

Throughout the afternoon, I took deep breaths to calm myself when the doctor wasn't looking. I told myself this wasn't personal; I had to learn the ropes.

At five o'clock, after eight hours of silence, I entered my car and burst into tears. Maybe my mother was right. Maybe I was too sensitive. Maybe I needed to grow up.

I returned the following week, pasting a smile on my face as I entered the waiting room. The receptionist didn't smile this time. She directed me to the exam room. Appointments had already started. Dr. Hoffman saw me and, wordless, pointed to the floor. I squatted on the mat next to the dog, bit my lip, and focused on the golden retriever.

Throughout the morning, Dr. Hoffman worked his magic. I had many questions, which I hoped he'd answer during lunch. When lunch break arrived, my enthusiasm bubbled out. "How do you know where to put the needles?" "How do you decide which herbs to use?" "What does 'triple-burner' mean?" I had jotted down the names of the supplements he'd prescribed to clients in a little spiral notebook.

"Don't worry about all that now," Paul said, scarfing down his hummus. "Wait until you take the course."

I didn't want to bother him, and I didn't want to eat, so I asked if he minded if I went through his medicine cabinet and wrote down the names of the herbs and vitamins he used, so that I could read up on them between sessions.

"Be my guest," he mumbled as he spread more hummus on a cracker.

I left the treatment-cum-lunchroom and headed to an overstuffed corner closet in the exam room. I scribbled down as many names as I could. Nothing meant anything to me, but I loved the fact the stuff was all natural, not a pharmaceutical in sight. The shelves of the stockroom at work, like all the hospitals I'd practiced at, were laden with poisons used for flea and tick prevention and dozens of prescription drugs with long fold-down inserts listing the many dangerous side effects in tiny print.

Toward the end of the day, I asked Paul if he could recommend any books. "Don't bother," he said. "If you want to do something, practice feeling a dog's body."

Huh?

"The depressions are all acupuncture points," he muttered.

I returned the next Wednesday hoping this opportunity would work out. The Wednesday proceeded like the others, except that as I was getting ready to leave, Paul laid out the terms of my future employment: I'd work under him, and he'd pay me ten dollars an hour.

He couldn't be serious. The vet techs at the hospital made more than that, and I'd been a licensed vet for six years! I stared at him, lost for words.

"I'll think about it," I sputtered.

I drove home in a daze. As soon as I entered my house, I called Mom. She knew how much this opportunity had meant to me.

"Why would you want to work for such a man? What could you possibly learn from someone like that?" Mom said. I told her I was learning this new way of healing. She said, "If you don't work for him, do you still want to take the course?"

I hadn't thought of that. I'd signed up for the IVAS course because I wanted to work with Hoffman and the course was a means to that end. I didn't want to start my own practice; I was not business oriented. I hated the money part of it, the managerial part, and the administrative part. I just wanted to help animals.

However, even though the acupuncture course was time-consuming, arduous, and expensive, it *could* change the trajectory of my professional life. Maybe this was the answer to my prayers.

Did I have the *chutzpa* to go it alone?

Chapter 32

"This Will Never Break"

In the meantime, Annie was still limping. Her gait and stance continued to be off, and I worried it would get worse. Dr. McCarthy in Darien had said she had a minor, soft-tissue injury but I was sure—and Hoffman had concurred—that she had a cruciate ligament tear. I called McCarthy for a follow-up.

Dr. McCarthy walked into the exam room, chart in hand, looking surprised. "What's going on with Annie?"

I paraded her up and down the hallway to demonstrate. "She looks fine," he said. I politely disagreed and insisted on an exploratory surgery. For me, surgery was the last option, but after three months of watching Annie limp, I felt the time had come. If we didn't stabilize the joint, the epiphysis (ends of the bones) would continue to rub against each other, causing osteoarthritis and life-long pain.

Reluctantly, he set a date and invited me to observe.

Hospitals admit surgical patients at an ungodly hour, but Dr. McCarthy generously allowed me to come around noon with Annie *NPO*, no eating or drinking after midnight. Anesthesia can cause vomiting, which can lead to aspiration pneumonia if food is inhaled into the lungs.

The receptionist directed us to the rear treatment area. Dr. McCarthy had a bad back, so I helped him lift Annie onto the stainless-steel table. He had me restrain her while he administered the anesthesia. I turned away as he inserted the needle. Then the techs took charge.

Dr. McCarthy, gowned and gloved, called me over. I peered into the drape as he cut.

"Well, well, well," he muttered, "look at this. The cruciate *is* partially torn. You were right." I sensed a new-found admiration. Given all that I'd seen and heard about Bill McCarthy from clients and vets over the years, I'd put him on a pedestal. Praise from him made my day.

"What does 'partial' mean, exactly?" I asked.

He pointed out the frayed white fibrous material of the anterior cruciate ligament which, together with the posterior cruciate, stabilizes the femur and the tibia. The anterior one takes the brunt of the trauma, he told me, and can fray over time, or it can tear in one fell swoop. "See, part of the ligament is still holding. Since it's not totally torn, Annie can still put weight on it. Look, the cartilage is smooth and healthy," he said.

Thank God.

I suddenly remembered what Dr. Hoffman and the immunologist from Cornell had told me. "Could you please biopsy her joint?" I told him about the auto-immune thing. He seemed skeptical but complied, and cut a small piece of tissue from the joint capsule. Then he removed a long piece of white nylon from the surgical pack.

"What's that?" I asked.

"Fishing line. Works great!"

He drilled a hole in the epiphysis of the femur and in the tibia. Then he pulled the fishing cord through and triple tied it "to stabilize the joint," he explained.

Whatever. I knew I was in good hands. I trusted McCarthy 100 percent.

Half an hour later, Annie began to wake up on a plaid blanket spread out on the surgery room floor. As soon as she struggled to stand, a tech helped me carry her to my car. Since I was a vet, they knew I could handle any post-op problems. When I stopped at the front desk to pay, the receptionist whooshed me out the door; McCarthy hadn't charged me a dime.

One week later, the animal hospital faxed me the results of Annie's biopsy, as I had requested. It came back positive for auto-immune disease. This meant that the rupture had most likely been caused by a vaccine.

I wondered how many other dogs had suffered the same fate as Annie?

Dr. McCarthy had told me to limit Annie to fifteen-minute leash walks for the first eight weeks of her recovery, and I followed his instructions. On the ninth week, Annie and I drove to the beach to celebrate. As a precaution, I kept her leashed. After we walked just a few minutes, Annie wouldn't budge. She held her right hind leg up in the air.

I tugged on the leash and convinced her to limp back to the car. Once home, I tried walking her slowly up the block. She hopped. She wouldn't put the leg down. With a sense of dread in my gut, I called the Darien Animal Hospital and begged the receptionist to get us in to see Dr. McCarthy as soon as possible.

A few days later we were back.

Dr. McCarthy looked concerned. "What happened?"

"I don't know. She won't put her leg down," I managed, barely controlling my anxiety. I told him we'd followed his instructions, and all had gone well, until I leash-walked her at the beach on week nine.

McCarthy examined Annie carefully, looking perplexed. He scheduled her for surgery the next day.

Dr. McCarthy opened her up in front of me and pulled out the severed line. "It seems the fishing line broke. This is a first for me." He seemed so genuinely upset that I didn't have the heart to get angry. I watched him manipulate Annie's knee, pushing the tibia forward of the femur. This was terrible, a *positive drawer sign* in vet lingo, confirming a complete tear. Dr. McCarthy apologized once again, still in disbelief, saying that he'd used a thickness more than enough for her eighty-five pounds. He asked the tech for an even thicker cord, "strong enough for a mastiff," he told me, adding, "This will never break."

Two months later her leg was up in the air once again. Recheck No. 2 with McCarthy. Same conclusion: another severed line. He was out of ideas.

I asked my bosses to recommend another surgeon.

Alan had heard good reports about a new guy in town, a Dr. Robert Miller. I immediately set up an appointment.

A cherub-faced man, who looked like he'd just graduated from high school, greeted me. His cheerful optimism put me at ease. I relayed Annie's history. When I reached the part about the fishing line, he grimaced. "I use wire. I've never had a problem with it," he said. The wire might eventually break, but the joint would remain stabilized, according to the doctor. "The broken wire can stay in her leg forever and not cause a problem," he said.

Annie's third surgery went well, but a few months later, she refused to walk. She held her leg at an odd angle when she was lying down and was clearly in pain. I examined her leg carefully. With my fingertips, I detected a piece of broken wire poking the skin, quite a distance from the knee joint. I caught my breath. The broken wire had migrated.

Back at his hospital, Dr. Miller looked bewildered.

This time, anger and frustration got the best of me. "I thought you said the broken wire wouldn't bother her!"

The doctor admitted Annie into the hospital for wire removal under anesthesia. Contrary to what he'd predicted, the knee joint hadn't held, either. Miller rewired her with a thicker gauge.

Chapter 33

A New Way to Heal

Annie seemed to be on the mend when the time came to fly to Atlanta for the first module of the International Veterinary Acupuncture Society's acupuncture course.

After breakfast, I retrieved my registration packet from the conference table and snuck into the meeting room an hour before lectures started. I grabbed my favorite seat—right front corner—just far enough away from the rest of the group to not be distracted and close to the speaker, but with the possibility of an easy escape if necessary.

I started to daydream in the large, airless conference room when a short, dark-haired woman sat down right next to me. *Really?* The whole room was empty!

Despite her invading my space, I reminded myself that I was here to connect with like-minded people. Small talk didn't come easily for me, but I pushed myself and started. "Hi, I'm Marcie. Looks like we're the first ones here."

Her name was Leslie, and she was from Houston.

"Do you have your own practice?" I asked.

"No, I work in a group practice three days a week, because I also work part-time at NASA."

NASA? That got my attention. "Really? What do you do there?"

"I'm a physicist."

"I'm impressed!"

"Don't be," Leslie laughed. "It's a lot easier than being a vet."

I asked why she was taking the course.

She told me that she'd been burning out (I could relate to that) until she took a seminar in animal communication that had re-energized her.

I'd never heard of an animal communicator, though I'd been to many psychics during my years in Italy. Each psychic had said that I would indeed graduate and predicted a professional future filled with love, but I never believed them. "Who gave the seminar?"

"Penelope Smith. She's incredible."

According to Leslie, Penelope had grown up in the Midwest, surrounded by cows. It seems the cows would describe their illnesses to Penelope, who'd pass the information along to the farmers, who'd then relay it to the veterinarians. The vets had been skeptical, but they listened, and the animals improved.

Man, I loved this kind of stuff!

"My colleagues at NASA laughed the whole thing off," Leslie said.

A year later, one of her NASA colleagues contacted her. The colleague's family had been murdered in their home, and the only witness had been the family dog. Remembering Leslie's story, the desperate colleague asked for the animal communicator's name and number. "Penelope 'spoke' with the dog," Leslie told me. "From the dog's description, they caught the murderer!"

The hairs on my neck stood up.

I'd never dare repeat this to my colleagues at my AVMA (American Veterinary Medical Association) or my CVMA (Connecticut Veterinary Medical Association) meetings. If I'd told my bosses at work, they'd probably reconsider my sanity, not to mention my aptitude for practicing medicine.

As Leslie and I spoke, the room filled with maybe a hundred vets from all over the States, peppered with a few foreigners, according to the list of attendees.

In the first lecture, I learned that acupuncture dated back eight thousand years to the Stone Age. According to the teacher, dogs had unearthed mummified humans that had the twelve acupuncture meridians tattooed on their bodies.

A medical textbook written around 2300 BC, the *Nei Jing* or *The Yellow Emperor's Classic of Internal Medicine*, was the bible of modern Chinese acupuncture. Using observation and practice only, as dissection was forbidden and anatomy unknown, the Chinese had discovered how to heal using meridians. These medical theories still held up, century after century.

Here, our medical protocols seemed to change at the drop of a hat, sometimes even doing an about-face. When I'd started working for the partners, I'd asked Alan about various treatment protocols. Why, for example, did we now use prednisone to treat pancreatitis, when I'd learned that prednisone could *cause* pancreatitis?

Alan told me about the old vet they'd bought the practice from. Seems the geezer had only two big bottles of medicine on his shelf: injectable penicillin and injectable triamcinolone (a long-acting steroid). He'd treated every disease with either one or both. Nothing else. The partners had made fun of him. Over the next twenty years, Alan and Mark had tried all the new drugs protocols. Alan chuckled. Maybe the guy had been right all along, he told me. Penicillin and steroids were probably all they really needed.

Here at the IVAS course, I entered an alternate medical universe, where medical interventions were based on the Eight Principles theory of Chinese medicine: Yin and Yang; interior and exterior; cold and heat; and deficiency (*xu*) and excess (*shi*). How interesting to view the world from this perspective! It appealed to me more than the lists of anti-this and anti-that drugs that caused all kinds of horrible side effects.

I recognized the word *Chi* (or *Qi),* but never really knew what it meant. The professor explained that *Chi* meant "life force" and said that it flowed along twelve meridians, in both humans and animals. Children are filled with Chi. Old people's Chi is waning. Chi is what differentiates being dead from being alive. A dead body has no Chi. This made sense.

When he began to speak about the meridians in relation to the *Zang-fu* organs (*huh?)* my eyelids grew heavy. I shook my head, unable to clear the fog. "*Zang-fu* organs produce and store *Chi* (energy), *Ji* (essence), and *Shen* (spirit)," the teacher said. I checked my watch—thirty minutes until break. I'd need more than the fruit and herbal tea they'd served at breakfast to stay awake.

When the teacher started in on the Five-Element Theory, something about the world being made up of wood, fire, earth, metal, and water, my mind shut down. I couldn't buy it. I couldn't even understand it. I hoped the practical part would be more relatable. I thumbed through our schedule. At least we'd have an equine and canine lab the next day.

During lunch break, things picked up. A Chinese girl, Wei Mei, joined me and a new friend, Cindy. Wei Mei practiced Reiki, a form of energy healing, and said she'd show us how to feel Chi. She had us rub our hands together hard and fast for a few minutes and then slowly pull them apart and bring them together again until we felt a ball of energy. She and Cindy seemed able to generate a sizeable ball. I had to try long and hard and several times to feel a two-inch diameter of the stuff between my palms. My energy ball was tiny because my Chi was low (no surprise, I don't sleep!). From an outsider's perspective, it probably looked as if we'd mimed it. But even though mine was small, I felt it: crinkly and crunchy. Fascinating!

The next morning, they divided us into two groups. Group One gathered outside for buses to the Equine Lab. I joined Group Two to the Canine Lab.

Several teachers were positioned around the classroom, each holding a leashed greyhound with black spots and numbers painted along the meridians of its body. I joined a cluster of students gathered around a tan greyhound. "Why do you use greyhounds?" I asked. The breed made perfect demonstration models, the teacher said, because of their short coats, clearly defined muscles, and docile natures. As we students poked and prodded, the instructor explained the dots and numbers. There were three hundred sixty-five acupuncture points, and we'd need to learn the bulk of them to pass our certification test. Of course, they wouldn't have us all stick needles into the dogs, but we'd need to indicate the points used to treat specific conditions.

Another exam? I'd thought I'd finished with exams after those fifty-one in vet school!

(For eight years, since leaving Bologna, I'd had nightmares that I hadn't finished my veterinary school exams and that I still had a dozen or so to go. I'd dream that the State Boards would find me out, and I'd lose my license. I'd wake up in a cold sweat.)

We switched venues after lunch. I boarded a bus to a stable. I had to stomp my feet to keep from freezing as the teacher demonstrated. Despite my love of horses, I thanked God that I'd gone into small-animal medicine—at least we practiced indoors, in the warmth.

By the time this first module was over, I couldn't wait to get home and try this new way of healing. I hoped to see some miracles.

Chapter 34

A Growing List of Miracles

I returned to work fired up, but kept my enthusiasm to myself. Out of nowhere, Mark invited me into his office and told me I could use the hospital during lunch and after hours to treat acupuncture patients. What a lovely and generous gesture! I looked for potential candidates each day during appointments. Hopeless cases with open-minded owners would probably be best. I offered my services free of charge, so what did they have to lose?

At the IVAS course, a professor had said that Intervertebral Disk Disease would be our "bread and butter." According to him, most of the dogs that were partially or totally paralyzed due to herniated disks responded to acupuncture. Though it had seemed unbelievable that a few needles could cure this crippling condition, I'd seen evidence first-hand during my stint with Dr. Hoffman. (Though I'd turned down the job offer, I remained grateful for all I'd learned there: both the miracles of acupuncture and the prospect of a 100 percent holistic practice.)

In the conventional world, corticosteroids helped some paralyzed dogs some of the time, but the animals almost always regressed. Surgery (to remove the diseased disk material, thereby relieving pressure on the spinal cord) was the treatment of choice. But it seemed that half of the time, surgery either didn't help or made the dog worse. Even though the owners had paid thousands of dollars in fees to the orthopedic surgeon, they got no guarantees.

Dachshunds are especially prone to ruptured disks, because of their long backs. Almost all develop back problems at some point in their life, and some of them end up paralyzed. I had seen many doxies strapped into carts, pulling themselves around by their front legs after an unsuccessful surgery. Most paralyzed dogs can't urinate without assistance. Over the years, I'd demonstrated to a dozen or so doxie owners how to manually express (empty) the dog's bladder. In addition, paralyzed dogs often developed fecal incontinence: poop would drop from their butts all over the house. It took an exceptional owner to manage this situation, and most of these dogs ended up euthanized.

I kept an eye out for injured dachshunds.

I didn't have long to wait. One day I met Mrs. G. in Room One with one of her three doxies. After examining the dog, I determined that Louie had stage-two disk disease out of a five-point grading scale. The dog was in a lot of pain but could walk with difficulty. He wobbled on his rear legs, like he was drunk. Both back legs had *conscious proprioceptive deficits*, meaning that when I placed a flexed paw on the table, Louie couldn't right it. Instead, he "knuckled," as he couldn't tell where his foot was in space.

Over the years, Mrs. G. had owned many dachshunds, some of which had had unsuccessful surgeries. She knew the drill: steroids or surgery. When I offered acupuncture as an alternative, she jumped at it. We set up an appointment for the next day. Becky, my favorite tech, agreed to help. All the techs at the hospital loved animals, but Becky had become my enthusiastic sidekick.

Come lunchtime the next day, Becky grabbed a towel from the laundry room and spread it on the slippery metal table. She stroked and reassured Louie while I did the proprioceptive test again. Same findings. I prepared the needles—long, pink-tipped needles for the deep musculature of the back, and short, half-inch blue-tipped needles for the less muscular knees and hocks.

First, I'd have to find the damaged disk. Mrs. G. had decided to skip the expense and invasiveness of the anesthesia needed for an X-ray, because we both knew radiographs often failed to pinpoint the diseased disk. MRIs could be useful, but also required anesthesia and were prohibitively expensive. Some of the instructors at IVAS had used the hand-friction technique to identify the bad disk. They'd rub their hands together to increase their

Chi, and then pass their hands slowly over the dog's back seeking heat, which indicated an injured disk. I tried but didn't succeed. My Chi was too weak.

But I didn't worry. In this new energic world, I felt like I was in *Godspace*. Healing didn't depend on me; my job was to allow God and His infinite power to work through me.

I pressed gently, but firmly, along Louie's bladder meridian, located on either side of the vertebrae, seeking the exact location of the injury. I knew that when I pressed on the damaged disk on his back, Louie would react, either by sinking, groaning, or even biting me.

The dog didn't flinch until I hit Bladder 21, the thoraco-lumbar junction, the vertebral space after the last rib, a common area for injury. Louie sank and groaned, a sure sign I'd located the correct spot. To be absolutely certain, I repeated my exam starting from the tail-end this time, instead of the neck. Sure enough, Louie sank and yelped at the exact same spot. A heck of a lot cheaper than an MRI!

Becky reassured the dog, while I readied the needles. Unlike when I handled scalpels, my hand didn't shake one bit. I inserted the pink needles in front of and behind the painful area. I put two more in back points that controlled ligaments and tendons. I placed a pink needle at the base of the neck and a corresponding one in the sacrum, opening up the flow of Chi to the whole spine. Louie looked worried but didn't move. Finally, I inserted a short blue needle in each hock, or ankle, which my teachers called the "aspirin point," the master pain point of the body. I put another in each knee, also points for ligaments and tendons. I stood back to assess my handiwork. Louie looked like a pincushion, but he seemed comfortable.

Next, I attached the leads from the brand-new, electro-stimulation machine that I'd bought at the conference. I told Becky to hold Louie while I ran to my office for the disposable camera that I'd brought in with me that morning. I snapped his picture.

I turned the machine on low. Louie stirred as he felt the tingling. Becky kept him still while I made sure the wires didn't fall off and pull the needles out with them. After fifteen minutes, I turned off the contraption and removed the needles. I had no idea how long the treatment took to kick in, or if it would even work.

I tested Louie's conscious proprioception again, by placing the top of one hind paw, then the other, on the table. Prior to my acupuncture treatment, Louie's feet had stayed in that unnatural position for at least six seconds. Normal is maximum two seconds. He now righted them immediately! Becky and I stared in amazement and then shared broad smiles.

Neither Alan nor Mark seemed at all interested in the outcome of my treatment.

Still, word spread. I started getting calls from dachshund owners from around the county. I'd occasionally treat the dogs during lunch break with Becky, but mostly I'd see them in the evening, after hours, with the owner assisting. The treatment itself took about half an hour. I'd see them once a week, and within six to eight weeks they were healed.

Healed!

A few months later, Mrs. G. brought in a second dachshund, Lucy. Lucy was totally paralyzed, without the ability to feel deep pain. I squeezed her toes with a hemostat as hard as I could, and she didn't react. Stage Five. The dog had been in this condition for at least five days: Too late for surgery and considered incurable. Mrs. G. had already brought Lucy to the orthopedic surgeon, who'd told her the dog would never walk again.

When Mrs. G. had called and asked if I could help, I told her I didn't know. But what did we have to lose? I saw Lucy twice weekly and treated her for free. Slowly, Lucy began to regain her ability to walk. After six weeks, she remained a little wobbly, like Louie had been. But not in pain. She reached 70 percent of normal, in my estimate. Not perfect, but for all three of us, another miracle.

One evening, a client returned with her black Lab mix for a second acupuncture treatment for the dog's severe arthritis. I couldn't put my finger on why, but he looked perkier than the last time I'd seen him.

"How is Chester doing?" I asked.

"Much better, Doctor. The most amazing thing happened. I never told you that my dog had been coughing every day for months. Chester hasn't coughed for a whole week! I can't believe it!" A look of astonishment spread across her face. "And his hair is growing back!" She showed me the area on his hip where he'd been shaved for a growth removal several months prior. "Look! See the stubble?"

I'd heard from other acupuncturists that unknown symptoms sometimes cleared up with seemingly unrelated treatment, and now I could see it for myself.

It seemed that the only side effect to acupuncture was curing other symptoms.

One afternoon, the receptionist told me that a client, Carolyn Lynch, was in Room One, asking specifically for *me* to recheck her sheltie, Shannon. This surprised me, because she usually saw Alan. I scanned Shannon's chart before I entered. Alan had diagnosed the dog with Inflammatory Bowel Disease (IBD) and had prescribed antibiotics and steroids.

"What's going on with Shannon?" I asked.

"I heard from a friend that you do acupuncture. Do you think it could help my dog?"

I told her that I'd learned in class that it could cure IBD, but that I'd never tried it.

"Could we try? I don't like the side effects of that prednisone." She rattled off a familiar list—drinking enormous amounts of water, losing control of his urine, agitation, ravenous appetite, weight gain, and hair loss.

She asked if I made house calls. I hadn't yet for acupuncture, but I jumped at the chance. I loved house calls. Entering someone else's world often felt like a mini vacation. She lived only ten minutes from the practice, so I had time for both a house call and Annie's walk during my two-hour lunch break.

I headed down a tree-lined driveway to her mansion. I'd felt clunky alongside Carolyn's refined and classy attire and manner, but I never imagined she had *this*. She steered me into a large, glassed sunroom where my patient awaited me. We lifted Shannon onto the rubber bath mat that Carolyn had placed on a mahogany table.

Six treatments later, Shannon was drug- and symptom-free: no more vomiting or diarrhea. His already luxuriant coat had grown even lusher. We scheduled a monthly maintenance plan.

With Shannon's IBD under my belt, I added acupuncture to my vaccine-oriented house-call-practice business cards.

Shortly afterward, I overheard a phone conversation between Alan and the local veterinary internal specialist, Dr. Fielding. Along with my bosses, I had referred many complicated cases to this guy over the years. From Alan's side of the exchange, I gathered they were discussing my use of acupuncture on dogs. When I questioned Alan, he snickered and told me that Dr. Fielding had said, "Anyone who claims they can successfully treat IBD with acupuncture is a quack."

A quack? I was stunned and hurt that Alan hadn't come to my defense—we had evidence! But I didn't say a word.

I soon added Max, a big white gentleman of a German Shepherd, to my growing list of acupuncture patients. Max, like many shepherds, had arthritis.

Annie and Max were dog park friends. Max's mom, Brenda, was one of those ladies from Westport who lunched and played bridge. Despite our different lifestyles, Brenda and I developed a close friendship. Skeptical about the side effects of the strong anti-inflammatories her regular vet had prescribed, Brenda had asked for my help. I supported her decision to stop the drugs and agreed to treat Max weekly at her home. The acupuncture worked: Max's mobility improved, he didn't limp, he showed no pain, and he ran around like normal.

Thanks to Brenda's extensive social network, my reputation and practice grew even wider.

One day, Alan brought in a boxer puppy from one of his pet stores. The ten-week-old pup had a case of severe generalized demodectic mange. A small number of demodectic mites normally live in the hair follicles and oil glands of dogs. If the dog's immune system is compromised, the mites proliferate, causing the hair to fall out. Veterinarians use various toxic injections, dips, and ointments to kill the mites. Mostly these drugs work, but sometimes they don't, and the dog remains hairless and covered with sores from secondary bacterial infections.

Conventional medicine held no hope for this puppy. Becky overheard Alan say that he planned to euthanize the dog. She ran to tell me, and we jumped into action. I had a gut feeling that acupuncture could heal the puppy, as his disease was a classic case of a poor immune system. Acupuncture works by strengthening the immune system, so maybe his body would fight off the mites better than with toxic chemicals. Again, we had nothing to lose—no owner, dog hopeless.

"Alan, would you mind if I tried acupuncture on the dog?" I asked. I didn't know if Alan would go for it. The dog was unsellable, and to maintain the pup in the hospital, Alan would have to pay for dog food, tech-time, and other expenses and inconveniences.

Alan shrugged. "Sure."

I said a silent prayer, grateful for the opportunity.

Becky shared my hope for a miracle for the puppy, which we named Rocco, and she agreed to help me with the treatments. Come noon, Becky placed the puppy on the metal exam table. Rocco was a sack of bones, head drooped, dejected and resigned.

I'd left my notes at home, so I scanned my mind, trying to remember the major immune boosting points. I recalled a few. I inserted needles between Rocco's dewclaw and his second toe, placed two in his back knees and a few along his back and hoped for the best. While we waited the twenty minutes needed to keep the needles in place, Becky and I discussed the horrors of pet stores, knowing full well that was our boss's sideline business. Then I pulled the needles out, and Becky placed Rocco back in his cage. With the whirlwind of activity in the hospital that afternoon, I left his care to the techs.

The next morning, I rushed to the boarding area to check my patient. Even in the cramped metal cage, I noticed a difference. Rocco's now bright eyes looked directly into mine. I reached in to stroke his head. "Rocco," I whispered, "you are my miracle dog. You will get better and better, don't worry."

I'd been taught that twice-weekly treatments were sufficient for most conditions, but I treated Rocco every single day. He was there. I was there. To my astonishment, his fur began to regrow rapidly. Where there'd been gray scaly skin, he now sported a shiny brown and white coat. Within a few weeks, he transformed into a normal, happy, energetic boxer puppy. Instead of ending up in the freezer with the other dead bodies, Rocco found a forever loving home, thanks to our rescue group, New Leash on Life.

I kept meticulous notes, as well as photos, of Rocco's miraculous transformation to use as my case study for certification.

Alan showed no interest in Rocco's progress. After he brought the puppy in, he never mentioned the dog again.

Apart from practicing my new skill, I'd had to prepare for quizzes and exams if I wanted my certification. Each night, after Annie's last walk, I'd sit cross-legged on my bed and study my notes until midnight. I didn't mind that my long days got even longer. I had a purpose and a goal: being a conduit for miracles, each treatment bringing me closer to God.

A year after I'd started, I flew to Atlanta for the last module and the certification test. I flubbed a few questions, but I passed. I was now one of about five hundred certified veterinary acupuncturists in the world.

I hiked my fee from zero to ten dollars a session.

Chapter 35

Parting Ways

In the following months, I scheduled acupuncture appointments during lunch breaks and evenings and house calls on weekends. My confidence grew with each success.

One morning, Simon, a dying fifteen-year-old setter mix, was admitted to the hospital. Simon hadn't eaten in days. We did the routine tests—blood work and X-rays—which came back normal. My bosses diagnosed him with "old age," a diagnosis I detested because in my opinion it was a cop-out. Alan suggested to the owner that we keep the dog in the hospital and give him IV fluids, injectable antibiotics, and an appetite stimulant for the next three days.

"If that doesn't work," Alan told him, "there's no hope." In other words, euthanasia would be the only option.

I watched Simon languish in his cage. Despite the drugs and IV, the dog hadn't eaten and in fact, hadn't moved. (Each time I passed his cage, I checked his breathing to make sure he was still alive.)

On the afternoon of the third and final day, I approached Alan. "Would you mind if I gave Simon an acupuncture treatment?" I had no idea if acupuncture could revive Simon, or if I had the necessary skill to help him, but I felt I had to try.

He glanced at his watch. "Do whatever you want. I'm putting the dog down in half an hour."

I ran to my office, grabbed two boxes of needles, and raced back to the dog. Simon lay sprawled on the metal floor of his cage, head pushed into

172

the corner, oblivious to me and to the commotion in the treatment room. I inserted needles into the strongest immune stimulating points I knew. The dog didn't flinch, not a whimper. Though dogs usually don't mind the needles, I would have welcomed any reaction. I crouched on the floor for about five minutes staring at him. My inner voice told me Simon needed more help. Divine help.

I had recently completed my first formal lesson in meditation. My teacher had spent many years working alongside the Maharishi Mahesh Yogi. I had tried for decades to meditate, but never had the patience. I willed myself to try again. I sat cross-legged in front of Simon, took his paw in my hand, and slowed and deepened my breaths. I emptied my mind, relaxed, and focused on allowing God's healing energy to flow through me, like a prism focusing light—through my head, down my arm, into my hand, and into Simon. I had never attempted anything like this; it simply felt like the right thing to do.

Within minutes, I literally felt an electric shock pass from my hand to the dog's paw, as if I'd put my finger into an electric socket. Simon and I jumped up in surprise, each of us with a little yelp. The techs came running. Simon sat up, eyes open and alert.

"Quick, get me a bowl of dog food!" I shouted. I watched, incredulous, as Simon gulped it down.

Alan entered the room, syringe loaded. He stared at Simon and the empty bowl. "Well, I guess I won't need the euthanasia solution," he said. And with that he moved on to his next appointment, never asking a thing about the treatment.

How could Alan ignore what he'd just witnessed with his own eyes? Hadn't he just deemed Simon's prognosis "hopeless" if the dog didn't respond to protocol? Wasn't the doctor even curious? Didn't he care? He'd conveyed similar disinterest in Rocco's healing, Shannon's healing, Louis' healing . . .

Alan had always been eager to teach me what *he* knew, and I soaked up his knowledge. Yet instead of being receptive to information from me that could save animals' lives, he seemed to ignore it. This was both disturbing and baffling.

I tried to dismiss these thoughts as I led Simon into Room One for his 5 p.m. discharge. Mr. A.'s face lit up with a broad smile, and I beamed as I handed him the leash. I wasn't going to tell him that I'd just performed a hands-on-healing and that God had healed his dog. I'd sound like some kind of woo woo. If I couldn't wrap my head around what I'd just experienced, how could I expect the owner to believe it? I told him I'd treated Simon with acupuncture instead.

That evening at home, as I lay in bed reflecting, a sense of awe filled me. I had no doubt that God had worked through me when I lay my hands on Simon.

When I returned to work, I couldn't wait to see what the new day would bring.

Alan seemed more distant than ever.

A short time later, I got an urgent call from Colette. She told me that the Connecticut State Legislature planned to vote on a "lemon law" for puppies from pet stores. The law stated that if a puppy became ill or died soon after purchase, the pet store would have to reimburse the owner the cost of the puppy, as well as the medical expenses incurred. Colette hoped that I, as the volunteer vet for our rescue group, would testify as an expert witness against the cruelty of pet stores.

Alan owned pet stores, and he knew how I felt about them. I'd seen first-hand how puppy mills treated those loveable, sentient creatures—as factory-made goods.

Yet speaking out against them publicly could jeopardize my job. "Let me think about it," I told Colette.

I loved my job. I'd finally found a hospital that practiced good medicine, run by veterinarians I respected. I'd put my heart and soul into my work for the past six years. At my age and pay scale, I knew it wouldn't be easy to find another position like this.

But my allegiance was to the animals. I had a voice, and I was learning to use it.

In the weeks leading up to the hearing, Alan and I didn't speak much. I suspected that Alan would show up to support a pet store's right to sell puppies, sick or not. I gathered he suspected I would speak out against them. I think we both knew what lay ahead.

After working all day at the hospital, I prepared my comments. Pet stores sold animals from those horrid puppy mills—places that churned out litter after litter from dogs kept in cramped cages in unsanitary and inhumane conditions. When the adults could no longer reproduce, they were killed. Pet stores are complicit in perpetuating this nightmare. Just like I'd done in Bologna, I wrote down the most important points on four-by-six index cards and then spoke them aloud to Annie, my audience of one. *Please, God, help me to let go of fear and have total faith in You!*

On hearing day, inside the gold-domed Connecticut State Capitol, I huddled with the other women from New Leash on Life. I reviewed the talking points on my index cards.

From the corner of my eye, I glimpsed Alan and Chris on the far side of the room, standing among other pet-store owners. The sight of them made me dizzy. I recognized some other veterinarians, too. Vets made a fortune off of pet stores. They visited the stores each week to vaccinate and treat sick puppies. In return, store owners referred new-puppy-owners back to those vets for a health check. Owners tended to use that same vet for the rest of their dogs' lives. Therefore, the more puppies the pet stores sold, the more clients the veterinarians acquired. *Quid pro quo.*

Alan noticed me from across the hearing room and stared. I tried to ignore him. I soaked up the righteous energy of my coalition. I practiced in my head, *"As a veterinarian of conscience, I feel it is my obligation to speak up against the inhumanity of puppy mills and the pet stores that enable them . . ."*

One by one people testified. I thought of all the sick puppies I'd treated from pet shops over the years and willed myself to ignore the men on the other side of the room, including my boss. I breathed deeply, calling on God for strength. And then—they concluded the hearing. They'd had enough testimony. No further comments. But the damage was done.

About three weeks later, late on a Friday afternoon, Mark and Alan called me into their office. Alan spoke, while Mark looked away.

"We think it's best we part ways," Alan said, his face blank and his tone expressionless. "Our philosophies are too different. You can stay on for a little while until you find another job."

I stared at the floor and tried not to cry. I knew that standing up for the dogs, which I'd pledged to do in the ashram in front of God, might lead to this. But being fired felt like a punch in the gut. I held back the tears until I reached my car.

For six years, this practice had been my life and my family. I had built my world around my job, even at the expense of a social life. And it had all been a big mistake.

I drove home to my two-room house, knelt on the floor, and hugged Annie, my rock. She still loved me. I wanted to call Mom, but then remembered what she'd said about Brenda, my dog-park friend. Brenda had left a job she loved to help her husband in his work. After thirty years of marriage, he left her for a younger woman, the latest in a string of affairs he'd had, she learned. When I'd told my mother that I was glad I hadn't wasted my life on a man and a lie, Mom had said that at least Brenda ended up with $1 million from the divorce settlement and two beautiful children. What did I have to show for my life, she wanted to know?

Now, after twenty years of studying and working, I had no money, no husband, no children, and no job.

It took all the courage I could muster to drive to work the next day. I felt like a beggar. I *was* a beggar. I lived paycheck to paycheck, and I needed this salary.

The sweet techs went out of their way to be nice to me, which made it worse. Before lunch break, Mark called me into his office and confided that firing me had not been his idea. He seemed so genuinely uncomfortable and looked so sad that I felt bad for him.

Alan ignored me and I him, as much as possible.

A few days later, I called my friend Rosemary, who always lifted my spirits.

"Pray to Baba," Rosemary said. "Something good will come out of this."

Something good? I didn't see how. But I did pray. Before bed, I held Baba's picture, the one I'd cut out of a book and framed more than fifteen years before, the one I'd prayed to before each and every exam. I knelt down by my bed and stared into Baba's eyes, which, as always, seemed to see straight into my soul.

"Baba, please help me. I can't do this on my own."

Chapter 36

Countdown to Aspen

The very next day the new AVMA journal arrived. I hadn't opened the classifieds in this magazine since Russell had fired me. I settled into my burlap-covered couch from the 1960s, a hand-me-down from my parents, with Annie at my feet and Shanti on my lap, tore off the plastic cover, and went straight to the help-wanted section.

A cursory scan revealed nothing within an hour's drive from my home. Upon closer inspection, I noticed an ad for an associate position an hour and a quarter away, but the job required emergency coverage. I'd sworn after leaving Russell's that I'd never work emergencies again. Exhausting and stressful, emergency calls obviated the possibility of any sort of a personal life. Even if I agreed to cover emergencies, the commute to the hospital could be a deal-breaker, as hospital owners want their associates close by. I called the hospital anyway.

I ignored the mileage and remained hopeful as I drove to Middlebury, cows dotting the pastures on either side of the highway. The sight of the black and white Holsteins relaxed me. Vet practice surely had to be more laid back in the country.

Dr. K hired me on the spot, agreeing that I wouldn't have to cover emergencies. I'd start in two weeks, which allowed me to give Alan and Mark the fortnight's notice I'd promised. *Thank You, God.*

The day before I was supposed to start, though, Dr. K called. He'd found a vet who lived close by and who could be on call for emergencies. In other words, I'd been hired and fired before I'd even started! Firing No. 4.

I grabbed Baba's picture from my dresser and stared into those eyes once again. And then, that very afternoon, my first copy of the *American Holistic Veterinary Medical Association Journal* arrived in the mail. I had joined the AHVMA after becoming certified in acupuncture, and the membership entitled me to their monthly magazine.

Two ads caught my eye. The first announced the annual holistic veterinary conference in Aspen, Colorado. Aspen sounded divine. Travel was my greatest joy, and I hadn't had time to travel for pleasure since beginning work as a vet eight long years before. The second eye-catcher promoted a course in classical homeopathy in Durham, North Carolina, given by a famous holistic veterinarian, Dr. Richard Pitcairn. (I even had his book!) Similar to the acupuncture course, the five modules would be given every two months. The course started in September, four months away.

Why not take it? With no job, I didn't need anyone's permission for time off. In fact, time loomed wide and empty into the foreseeable future, a terrifying thought. I needed structure for my mental health. A bimonthly timetable would keep me focused and punctuate my life with something to look forward to for an entire year.

I knew very little about homeopathy. I'd bought a book on it from a health food store during my freshman year of college, but I couldn't make it past the first chapter. Lots of Latin names with numbers and something to do with healing with energy. I'd found it weird and confusing. Yet ever since the acupuncture course, I knew alternative medicine was my path. Already, I felt that acupuncture was not enough; I wanted to expand my repertoire. Homeopathy could be another tool in my toolbox.

I learned that a local veterinarian practiced homeopathy, and I contacted him. I spent a couple of days observing Dr. Warner in his Greenwich hospital, hoping to witness the miracles of homeopathy. Instead, I saw the doctor and a client celebrate the resolution of her dog's ear infection after twelve months of treatment. Both doctor and client were ecstatic. Were they kidding? One week of antibiotics would've done the trick.

Still, this professional homeopathic course for veterinarians beckoned. I had the time. All I needed was the money to pay for it.

Spiritual people say that when something is meant to be, things fall into place.

Out of the blue, I received a call from an old colleague. I'd met her almost a decade earlier in New York City, while I was living with Grandma and studying for the boards. She asked if I could fill in for her at a Yorktown Heights veterinary hospital, located about an hour from my home, while she went on vacation. The hospital needed a relief vet for two weeks. I'd never heard of short-term positions. She said they paid thirty-five dollars an hour. That was more than I'd ever earned. A windfall!

A few days later, I drove to Yorktown Heights and interviewed with the two elderly partners over frozen yogurt at a local mall. They didn't seem to care that I didn't do surgery. In fact, they didn't seem to care about anything other than their extra-large portions of chocolate yogurt dripping with multiple toppings. When I confessed my insecurity of running their hospital alone, they shrugged. They told me that I could refer difficult cases to another practice or to the local emergency hospital. They asked me how I liked the yogurt.

That evening, filled with hope and anticipation, I completed my applications for both the Aspen conference and the homeopathy course.

During my two-week relief vet gig in Yorktown, I hung out with the techs and chatted. With no boss breathing down my back, no jealous co-workers, and only an occasional client, I felt like I'd hit the jackpot!

A few per-diem jobs at other hospitals later, I realized that despite my minimal surgical skills, I could make a decent living doing this work. Empowered and optimistic, I signed a twelve-month contract at a local gym and even decided to buy a house, things I'd avoided out of fear of getting fired. Grandma had left me just enough money for a small down payment on an inexpensive house. I wanted a place where I could live *and* work, as I couldn't afford an office space to build my not-yet-existent holistic practice.

Mom drove up from Lido to house-hunt with me. We found a just-barely affordable fixer-upper near my Fairfield rental. The realtor assured us that I could practice medicine out of the house.

Things seemed to be falling into place. I interviewed for three steady part-time jobs and all three hospitals wanted me. I accepted them all. I told everybody in advance about my homeopathy course. "No problem," they said, "we'll work around your schedule."

In Oxford, I worked two days a week out of a converted barn, red with a silo. It felt absolutely bucolic—until I stepped inside. The place was a madhouse, with two or three receptionists and minimum of four or five techs. There were three of us vets: the owner, a short intense man, who paid me little heed; Dr. Giordano, an associate around my age, who'd worked there for years (and loved surgery); and me.

My appointments, scheduled at ten-minute intervals, felt like an assembly line. Since most appointments were healthy animals in for vaccinations, ten minutes usually sufficed. I approximated forty-five patients during my eleven-hour day.

I had no formal lunch hour. Instead, I slipped into the narrow communal kitchen during appointments where I choked down my cheese sandwich and helped myself to Mr. Coffee, which caffeinated me all day.

The boss kept small metal trash containers in each room, where the staff tossed everything, including excised pet body parts—ovaries here, testicles there—without springing for plastic trash bags.

The second hospital was a small, one-man practice in Fairfield. I'd heard good things about Dr. Hunter over the years from his clients, including Rosemary. He'd treated her fourteen-year-old miniature schnauzer, Bandit, for advanced liver disease and heart failure. The dog hadn't responded to his treatment, though, so Dr. Hunter had told Rosemary that euthanasia was the only option.

Rosemary had brought Bandit home to die, but before planning his funeral she called me to see if I could help. I didn't know, I told her. I gave him an acupuncture treatment and then went home. Apparently, the previously anorectic and dying dog then ate a pound of roast beef. He continued to improve so much that Rosemary called Hunter to cancel the euthanasia appointment and told him the good news.

It seems Hunter had been impressed, because soon after, he called to ask me if I was interested in a part-time job on his day off.

Dr. Hunter didn't give a hoot about my lack of surgical skills. He told me he'd come in for any emergency surgery, and the rest could wait. He encouraged me to use his office in the evenings for my personal acupuncture clients. Impressed with his openness to acupuncture and his apparent lack of ego, I accepted.

My days there were pretty boring, as most of his clients waited to see him. I avoided the snarky tech and hung out in the doctor's office reading through his stack of old journals.

The third hospital reminded me of my old job in Queens. Located in a rough neighborhood in West Haven, my day was filled with botched, home-cut tail dockings, injured pit bulls (probably from fights), and unvaccinated puppies, often sick.

The staff mirrored the clients. I'd watch, fascinated and unnerved, when techs restrained fractious cats in the treatment area by hogtying the felines to wooden planks, like a bull in a rodeo. While the cats' eyes dilated into black pools of fear, the techs calmly drew blood, bathed, shaved, or did whatever else needed to be done. Other hospitals would have anesthetized these mini tigers, but perhaps Dr. Young wanted to avoid the risk of anesthesia. When I thought about it, which I tried not to, the method was brilliant, though disturbing.

Somehow, my schedule worked out well. Just when I thought I couldn't take one place anymore, it was time to move along to the next.

In the meantime, I counted down the days to Aspen. In August, after a short stay with a third cousin in Denver, I boarded a small propeller plane to the famous ski-resort town. A middle-aged woman in the seat next to me introduced herself: "Hi, I'm Jean. Are you going to the conference?"

How could she tell I was a vet? True, I could usually pick out veterinarians from other guests at hotel-hosted conferences, thanks to our dowdy clothing, sensible shoes, and no makeup. Did I really look so boring?

"Yeah," I mumbled, trying not to feel insulted. "You?"

She smiled. "I've been speaking at these conferences for years."

"You're a lecturer?"

"I'm an immunologist. I'll be speaking about vaccines."

She seemed nice enough. We exchanged a few more pleasantries. After we landed, I checked into the hotel, ordered room service, and went straight to bed. I wanted to get up early to grab my favorite seat in the lecture hall.

The multi-tiered conference room soon filled with over a hundred people. I watched, stunned, as Jean walked on the stage.

Chapter 37

Cause and Effect

I whispered to the woman beside me that I'd sat next to the lady on the stage on my flight from Denver.

"Are you kidding?" she said. "You know Jean Dodds?"

I learned even more about this extraordinary woman, Dr. Jean Dodds, the top veterinary immunologist in the world, during the next hour and a half as she shredded the AVMA's vaccine protocols. I sat riveted. Dr. Dodds asserted that we over-vaccinate our companion animals and condemned vaccines as the principle cause of auto-immune disease. This was exactly what the vet-immunologist from Cornell had told me! Dr. Dodds explained that many of the so-called idiopathic diseases—meaning diseases from unknown causes—are actually auto-immune diseases, which occur when the body's immune system mistakenly attacks and destroys its own tissues and organs.

Many of the ailments I'd treated, including allergies, hypothyroidism, rheumatoid arthritis, degenerative myelopathy, dry eye, inflammatory bowel disease, Addison's disease, Cushing's disease, and dozens of others, she attributed to vaccinations. I followed her every word, taking notes and attempting to absorb the information.

My brain went into overload. In my life, I must have administered thousands of vaccines—probably ten thousand—for canine distemper, feline distemper, feline leukemia, Lyme, rabies, and kennel cough, including to my own dogs and cats.

I'd always prided myself on being able to differentiate fact from fiction, but this didn't make sense. How was it possible for all of these diseases to be caused by vaccines? It seemed ludicrous. And yet, Dr. Dodds's humility, her apparent love for animals, and her data-driven, evidence-based science made it difficult *not* to believe this.

Dr. Dodds gained nothing from advising against vaccines. We veterinarians, on the other hand, rode a financial wave powered by yearly vaccine protocols dictated by pharmaceutical companies. Not only that, but most of our income came from treating diseases *caused,* Dr. Dodds maintained, by those very vaccinations, creating a self-propagating circle.

All day long, I ruminated on this new information. At night, as I attempted to fall asleep, I thought of all the pets, beloved by myself and my clients, that I'd vaccinated.

Had I, who loved animals, betrayed them?

The next day, after lunch, I joined our group for a bus tour. As shimmering yellow Aspen trees raced by my window, I fell into a contemplative state. Forty minutes later, we pulled over and exited the bus to take in the view. I lost myself in the beauty and grandeur of the golden mountains. A sense of myself as a separate, anxious entity faded as I merged into the vastness that surrounded me.

A veterinarian's life is fraught with pressure. With constant life and death decisions, nervous and angry clients, and hectic seventy-plus hour work weeks, it's no surprise we have one of the highest suicide rates among professionals. Admittedly, I hadn't coped so well over the years. The friendly techs in West Haven had given me the affectionate nickname "Dr. Panic."

But there, among the Aspens, as my breathing deepened and peace permeated me, I questioned whether I could continue to work in the conventional veterinary world. My job was to follow hospital protocol, not to decide whether or not to vaccinate. That wasn't my call.

And my thriving house-call business—essential to my financial survival—was based almost exclusively on vaccines.

As intelligent and credible as this Dr. Dodds seemed, the New Yorker in me remained skeptical. Hearing was one thing, but seeing *evidence* was believing. I returned to work in Connecticut, determined to keep a close eye on the animals I'd vaccinated.

Clients at the busy Oxford practice ran the gamut. Some responded enthusiastically to yearly vaccine reminders, which the receptionists plastered with Post-its on each animal's file. Pre-Aspen, I'd embraced the party line and tried to convince the owners to get every single one. I'd cite the many contagious diseases that lurked about and could sicken or kill their cats and dogs. Now, Post-Aspen, I asked *which* vaccines they wanted. I felt a bit weak in the knees when they said they wanted them all—especially if their animal was old or sick.

What if vaccines hit those animals the hardest, as Jean Dodds warned?

I paid closer attention to our old-timer clients, especially those who reluctantly brought in their pets for annual vaccinations. Many said that they'd not taken their previous dogs in for yearly vaccinations, and *they'd* lived into their late teens—with rarely a visit to the vet. Now, they said they were "always here" and their animals were "always sick."

Pre-Aspen, I didn't give this much thought. Now, I wondered whether they were onto something.

The third type of client in Oxford—farmers who treated their pets like livestock—would bring in their dogs and cats only when injured. These animals hadn't been to a vet in years, yet they seemed to be the healthiest. Once the owners were in our door, we pushed every possible vaccine, shaming the owners into compliance. Now, though, I needed evidence. I started to notice a few things. Days to weeks after being vaccinated, many pets would come back with some ailment or another: an ear infection, a skin allergy, seizures, even cancer. "You missed my dog's ear infection!" one client told me a week after I gave the spaniel his distemper shot. In the past, mystified, I'd probably have blamed myself for an oversight. But now, with Dr. Dodds's lecture hitting home, I wasn't so sure.

I'd shared what I'd learned from Dr. Dodds with the techs. They seemed skeptical too. But soon, they began bringing cases to my attention.

"Marcie," one sweet tech at Oxford said, "someone just brought their dog back for seizures. She was totally healthy a couple of days ago when Doc gave her a rabies vaccine."

Her colleague chimed in. "Since you told me, I've been checking the records before I put clients in the exam room. So many animals come back with ear infections, diarrhea, and other stuff after their shots. I can't believe it!"

After a couple of months of this, armed with my anecdotal evidence and Jean Dodds's years of research, I sought out my boss, certain he'd want to know. He'd surely be horrified, same as me. Instead, after I shared the information with him, he shot me a piercing look and turned on his heel.

At the West Haven practice, it was not unusual for owners, often of pit bulls or Rotties, to delay their puppy shots. They'd often brought in older pups—twelve-weeks old, not the recommended eight weeks—for their first shots. Within a day or so post-vaccine, however, some had returned with sick puppies.

"That's because you didn't bring them in earlier," I'd chastise them. "The dog must've been harboring something."

This was what the hotline of a pharmaceutical company had expressly told me to say. During a house call, I'd convinced a woman to vaccinate her perfectly healthy, outdoor, six-year-old domestic short-hair cat for feline leukemia. That was the only thing I administered. The next day the woman called to tell me her cat was vomiting and wouldn't eat a thing. I raced back, drew blood from the cat, and sent it to the lab. The bloodwork indicated the cat was in kidney and liver failure. I called the pharmaceutical company to report an adverse reaction. The pharmaceutical rep told me that the failing kidneys and liver had nothing to do with their vaccine. "The cat must've been harboring something," the rep said. "Tell them that."

I didn't believe them then, and now those words rung in my ears. Maybe vaccines weren't about science, but about money. Big money.

Had Dr. Dodds's conclusions been staring me in the face for years, but I hadn't connected the dots?

Not long after, the *Danbury News Times*, a local newspaper, called. They wanted to interview me for a story on acupuncture. I don't know how they'd heard about me. I'd been certified just one year and had treated only about a hundred animals. The reporter wanted to do the story ASAP, with photos.

She arranged to interview me at my home and agreed to use Annie for the pictures. I lined up clients available for phone interviews. Soon after, the *Connecticut Post*, one of the largest newspapers in the state, wrote a story on me.

Then Channel 12, the local Connecticut TV station, inquired. They wanted to film me for a half-hour segment on acupuncture. Though being in front of a camera terrified me, I believed Divinity was at work. This could be my passport to my true calling. I said I'd do it.

I wanted the perfect client and patient, so I asked my friend Brenda, whose arthritic shepherd, the calm and photogenic Max, seemed ideal for TV. Brenda was not at all camera shy and loved to brag about Max's success with acupuncture. Plus, her Westport mansion would make a lovely backdrop.

After the articles and TV show, my phone started ringing off the hook. But the callers would have to wait. I was heading to Durham, North Carolina, for Dr. Pitcairn's Professional Course in Classical Homeopathy.

Chapter 38

Roadkill for Dinner

In the pre-conference breakfast hall, I bypassed the baskets of herbal teas and hot water and filled a white mug from the single coffee urn. I slipped a couple of honey cluster raisin bars into my purse and then turned to check out the attendees. Most seemed to be women in their early forties, around my age, wearing friendly faces.

Dr. Pitcairn ("call me Richard") welcomed us with a smile from the podium. He began by telling us how he'd begun his holistic journey: after vet school, he'd worked at a busy mixed animal practice (both large and small animals) but saw that many of his patients didn't improve with the recommended protocols. He resolved to do better. Five years and a PhD in veterinary immunology later, he said he'd hit a "medical dead end."

Undeterred, he began a deep dive into nutrition. He, like me, hadn't learned a thing about nutrition in vet school. We vets repeated what our veterinary elders and the pet food reps had said: feed a good commercial diet (preferably the ones we sold) and avoid table scraps. But Richard was wary. In the past, he'd worked in a chicken-butchering factory in Maine, where USDA trimmers and inspectors worked upstream from him on the conveyer belt, tossing diseased and damaged parts of the chickens into metal drums. These were deemed unfit for human consumption and were sent to pet-food factories instead.

Richard said that pet foods—both store brands and vet endorsed—included "the 4-Ds": dead, diseased, disabled, and dying animals sourced from slaughterhouses; road kill; *even euthanized dogs and cats* from shelters (euthanasia solution included). Plus, the antibiotics, herbicides, pesticides, drug residues, and toxic heavy metals found in and on the animals.

Instead, Pitcairn maintained, dogs and cats should eat as their wild cousins ate—as wolves, foxes, lions and tigers did. "Predators eat prey." In other words, raw flesh, organ meat, bones, and the grassy intestinal contents of their herbivore kill.

Raw meat. Even the idea made me queasy, especially because I'd been a vegetarian for so long.

According to the doctor's research, 70 percent of commercial dry dog foods contain salmonella (bacteria), which could cause vomiting and diarrhea and other problems. True, there are many types of bacteria (usually harmless) in dog poop, but Richard had not encountered any sickness due to bacteria, salmonella or otherwise, in his years of prescribing a raw diet. This made sense—as gross as it seems, dogs eat their own and others' poop and lick their butts all the time with no problems! As for cats, Richard cited a study that found cats' health plummeted and mortality skyrocketed when cats ate cooked meat from restaurant leftovers. The trajectory reversed when they returned to a raw-meat-based diet.

After lunch, Richard dove into the topic of vaccines. As a veterinarian with a PhD in immunology, he'd considered vaccines sacrosanct, just as I had. Though I'd distrusted pharmaceuticals, what with all those pages of warnings and side effects, until Dr. Dodds's lecture I'd never doubted that vaccinations were safe and effective. But I thought about the pharmaceutical companies' many booths at our continuing education conferences and realized these were the very companies sponsoring many of the events. My bosses powwowed with pharmaceutical reps on a regular basis. My thinking, I realized, was shaped by this skewed perspective.

Richard offered a different point of view. A vaccine's efficacy depended on the state of the animal. If an animal was too young, too sick, or too weak or malnourished, it couldn't mount a proper immune response to a vaccine. An existing disease, or concurrent medication, such as steroids, could undermine the immune system's response to a vaccine. And anesthesia depressed the immune system for weeks. For convenience sake, all the hospitals I'd worked in routinely administered vaccines while animals were under anesthesia—while being spayed or neutered, or whatever. This could include a canine distemper shot (which included five different viruses), the kennel cough vaccine, the Lyme vaccine, and the rabies vaccine. That could be nine vaccines at once! With or without the anesthesia, we'd administer *all* the vaccines together, every single year. And the more vaccines we gave, the more it compromised the immune system, Richard's research showed.

(At least in the hospitals where I'd worked, we never vaccinated pregnant animals. We'd all learned in vet school that was a big no no, as it caused miscarriages and congenital abnormalities to the fetus.)

The small print in vaccine inserts listing possible side effects were only the "tip of the iceberg," Richard said. He blamed vaccines for the bulk of chronic disease in our patients, just as Dr. Dodds had. While vaccines usually prevented the acute viral form of a disease, they often substituted a more pernicious, chronic form of disease into the animal, Richard reported. Plus, as harsh as it sounds, the acute viral form has a purpose: to strengthen the species. As a virus sweeps through the population, it kills off the weakest of the herd, ensuring "the survival of the fittest."

My head began to swim. Thankfully, tea break was announced.

While we queued up for goodies, I chatted with the blonde ahead of me. Somehow the subject of God came up. I mustered the courage to tell her I'd been a Sai Baba devotee for fifteen years, a fact I'd never mentioned to other vets, even to my acupuncture colleagues.

"My brother is a devotee also," she said, as if it was the most natural thing on earth. "He's been to India several times."

This was the first non-Indian I'd met in America who had even heard of Sai Baba. I couldn't believe I was with veterinarians where I could be myself.

Back to the seminar. We had been taught in vet school that immunity stemming from a natural disease and immunity due to a vaccine were more or less equivalent. Richard's evidence showed otherwise. He used measles, the human equivalent of canine distemper, as an example. "We contract measles by breathing the virus into our mouth or nose, the natural route of transmission, so the virus first comes into contact with our regional lymph nodes, which produces a local immune response," he said. To protect the body from systemic organ damage, the lymph nodes stimulate the production of specific local antibodies, mobilizing white blood cells and chemical mediators to fight the intruding germ.

But vaccines bypass those local defense systems. They enter the bloodstream via an injection and spread throughout the body. Our immune systems are not built to deal with this unnatural assault, he told us. As a result, the body can get confused and overreact to the invading foreign substance, attacking its own tissue along with the antigen in the vaccine. This is what creates auto-immune diseases.

Richard rattled off a list of common vaccine-induced diseases: inflammatory bowel disease, allergies, asthma, arthritis, paralysis, seizures, encephalitis, lupus . . . These conditions take days to weeks to fully develop, so veterinarians don't connect the diseases to the vaccines, he said.

Who knew? I slumped in my seat. Thank God, dinner break was announced.

Chapter 39

Risks vs. Benefits

Early the next morning, I wandered into the hotel's breakfast room, where I recognized some attendees and asked if I could join them.

"Of course," said a freckled-faced woman. Turned out, she and another vet, originally from South Africa, practiced in Florida near where my parents, now snowbirds, had a second home. We talked non-stop. (I made a mental note to tell my mom and dad to transfer their cats' care to one of those hospitals.) We had much in common: shared histories of professional burnout and mid-life crises, combined with hopes for a new beginning.

Folks here seemed different from even the acupuncture vets, where a streak of ego ran through many of the lecturers and students that I'd met. Acupuncture had a sort of macho cowboy mentality. (Someone at the table who had also taken the IVAS course joked that acupuncture was the holistic equivalent of orthopedic surgery.) With acupuncture, you *did* something: you stuck a needle in, you attached electrodes, and turned on electricity. Since all meridians are connected, wherever you put the needle, something positive seemed to happen.

I'd accomplished that without having to think too hard. Homeopathy, as I was about to learn, took dedication and hard work, as well as about twenty years' practice and lots of study. There was no room for ego and, without quick fixes, not much money to be made, either.

Laurie, Richard's pretty young associate, presented the first lecture of the day. A conventionally trained vet, like all of us, she had accompanied her husband, a wildlife vet, on hundreds of rounds to investigate dead wildlife out west where they lived. The animals had died in perfect health, either by car or gunshot. No allergies, ear infections, arthritis, warts. Nothing. "Not a single carcass displayed any sign of chronic disease," Laurie reported. "That was my aha moment."

I thought about the hundreds of squirrels I'd seen smushed on the street while walking my dogs. Even though I'd observed fleas in their fur, not a single squirrel had flea allergy dermatitis or anything else marring their perfect flattened bodies. Nor had I noticed hair loss or growths or anything abnormal on the dead opossums, raccoons, or deer that littered the sides of Connecticut's roads.

Were we doing something to our pets that caused many of their problems?

Laurie thought so. Like Dr. Dodds, she attributed most of the maladies we saw in our practices to vaccines, calling them "the worst thing we inflicted on our pets."

By now, I had vaccinated thousands of animals in my years of practice.

After Laurie's lecture, Richard took to the podium and referred us to our handouts, specifically to an excerpt from the conventional veterinary bible, *Current Veterinary Therapy (XI)*.

He read, "A practice that was started many years ago and that lacks scientific validity or verification is annual revaccinations. *Almost without exception there is no immunologic requirement for annual revaccination.* Immunity to viruses persists for years or for the life of the animal. Successful vaccination to most bacterial pathogens produces an immunologic memory that remains for years. . ."

In other words, where viruses are concerned, it's like the polio vaccine. It lasts a lifetime. In the case of a bacterium, like tetanus, the vaccine lasts about ten years.

The only rationale for annual vaccines, the authors concluded, was to get the animals in for an office visit to increase income. Richard suggested that we vets needed to understand *vaccinosis*—vaccine-induced disease in order to treat the chronic diseases that constitute the bulk of our practice. He asked us to envision a rabid dog. This was easy: vicious, foaming mouth, staring eyes, staggering. Rabies paralyzes the throat muscles, impeding swallowing, and saliva gathers and drips from rabid dogs' mouths. With rabies vaccinosis, he said we'd see similar, attenuated symptoms, like laryngeal paralysis, reverse sneezing, chronic drooling, sloppy eaters and drinkers, and dogs that can't tolerate collars around their necks—or even hugs.

Rabid dogs (or other rabid animals), undergo a personality change as well. They can lose all fear, become aggressive, and be driven to bite and kill.

"Think of some of your canine patients. I'm sure you've all seen dogs that are suspicious and aggressive to strangers, uniformed people, or other dogs. This is *not* normal behavior," Richard said. He attributed this behavior to the rabies vaccine. "Many symptoms we see are so common that we think they're normal. But they're not."

I'd seen many dogs dropped off at shelters, or euthanized, for aggression. How heartbreaking to think these deaths could have been avoided.

As Richard spoke, my mind wandered. Often, clients would ask what caused this or that symptom. Often, I didn't have a clue. I'd admit that I didn't know, although this embarrassed me. My bosses, though, either ignored the question or made up something I *knew* wasn't true.

On the other hand, they *did* acknowledge that the recent rash of fibrosarcomas in cats was caused by the rabies vaccine, and occasionally by the leukemia vaccine. Fibrosarcomas were historically rare. And fatal. Lately, these tumors were popping up more and more at the injection site of a vaccine, typically administered in the scruff of the neck. Despite aggressive surgery, the tumors always recurred. As a result, the American Veterinary Medical Association recommended that we instead administer the rabies shot in the right thigh, and the leukemia shot in the left—that way we could amputate a leg if a tumor appeared. (When we'd heard about this recommendation during my time with the two partners, Alan had joked that we should inject the vaccine in the tail—better to lose a tail than a leg. I had thought that a brilliant idea.)

Richard believed that we should conduct a risk-versus-benefit evaluation for each vaccine for every animal and that a vaccine should be considered only if the disease had a high mortality rate *and* the animal had a high likelihood of exposure. So, an indoor cat, for example, should not need a feline leukemia vaccine because the virus was transmitted by close contact with infected cats.

The same risk-versus-benefit standard should be applied to re-vaccination, he said. If you administer a puppy or kitten shot at sixteen weeks old, more vaccines rarely enhanced immunity, the studies showed. Instead, more vaccines led to more vaccine-induced disease.

Why continue to vaccine, Richard said, when tests exist to measure an animal's immunity? When we vaccinate an animal, we introduce an antigen (a weakened form of the virus or bacteria) into the animal's body. The antigen stimulates an immunity to the same germ, in the form of antibodies. With a simple blood test, laboratories can measure the quantity of antibodies, called "titers," circulating in an animal's blood. An adequate titer confirms that an animal is likely protected from a particular disease and doesn't need another vaccine.

While I worked for Alan and Mark, a client brought in a black cat that was acting strangely. The cat had never been vaccinated for rabies and had been mauled by a raccoon several days earlier. Per protocol, my bosses caged the cat in the treatment area for observation. After the ten-day waiting period, we (they) euthanized the cat, cut off its head, and sent it to the state lab to test for rabies. The test came back positive. The techs, who had handled the cat, received post-exposure antibody injections, plus a rabies vaccine. The other docs and I just got a rabies vaccine.

The state told us to follow-up our vaccine in a year, either with a booster shot or an antibody titer test.

The following year, I overheard Mark and Alan setting up a blood titer test for themselves in lieu of the shot. I asked if I could get one also, and they agreed. My titer came back sixty times the required level for protection—meaning it would most likely suffice for the rest of my life. The rest of the staff hadn't been offered the option of the titer test because the booster vaccine was cheaper.

A few weeks later, I overheard some of the girls, including my sweet sidekick Becky, discussing recent ailments they'd all had—mostly joint pain. The girls thought they'd contracted Lyme disease. But I remembered their recent booster and told them to check out the vaccine insert. The listed side-effects mirrored their symptoms.

Here at the conference, Richard explained that vaccines target a particular breed's genetic weak point. I remembered an article I'd read in the veterinary journal *Compendium* about Degenerative Myelopathy (DM), a dreaded auto-immune disease that attacks the spinal cord of primarily German Shepherds and Shepherd mixes. It's the canine equivalent of multiple sclerosis. Over the course of six months to a year, the dogs' legs gradually become paralyzed. My heart sank when I'd see these dogs stumble into the exam room. I knew the diagnosis straightaway. With DM, the dogs felt no pain and dragged themselves around without discomfort. (The other possibilities were Intervertebral Disk Disease and spinal tumors, but those things were painful.) There is no cure for DM.

According to the *Compendium* article, researchers had isolated the distemper antigen from the spinal cords of euthanized dogs with DM. They discovered that the dogs hadn't been sick with distemper; rather, the DM stemmed from the distemper vaccine.

Now I understood. German shepherds are notorious for rear-end weakness, which evidently is their genetic weak link, so this predisposed them to the neurological form of distemper vaccinosis.

Finally, Richard introduced homeopathy. The crucial difference between conventional medicine and homeopathy, he said, is that conventional medicine merely aims to stop symptoms. In conventional treatment (or allopathy, derived from the Greek root *allo*, meaning "other"), doctors administer drugs that work in opposition to the symptoms. For example, if a dog has a fever, an allopathic vet will administer anti-febrile drugs.

Homeopathy (*homoios*, meaning "similar") understands that the body knows best and simply needs an "assist" in its attempt to heal. A fever is an inflammatory response generated by the body in its attempt to heal itself (e.g. from an invading virus). A homeopathic doctor uses remedies derived from things like plants and minerals that work *with* the body to fight off the invading germ, rather than work *against* the body. The homeopathic remedies act as catalysts to help return the individual to homeostasis (equilibrium or health).

Most conventional Western medicine doesn't cure disease; it simply palliates or suppresses symptoms. With *palliation*, drugs might rid the body of the symptoms. But when the medicine is discontinued, the same symptoms eventually return, though sometimes in a different location, and sometimes worse. With *suppression*, the drug stamps out the offending symptom, but drives the disease deeper in the body, creating a more serious disease.

Allopathic medicine lumps symptoms of patients into easily defined categories so they can all be treated by the same drug or drugs. A conventional vet might diagnose "allergy" for all itchy dogs, for example, and administer prednisone with all its unwanted side-effects. We always gave steroids to itchy dogs and cats. Sometimes we recommended allergy testing to see what the animal was allergic to. But why had the cat or dog developed the allergy in the first place? Didn't matter.

Homeopathic doctors are like detectives in their quest to uncover the *root* of a disease. Finding the cause helps determine the cure. Cure means the body is healed and needs no further treatment.

If a homeopathic vet suspects an itchy patient's symptoms are caused by a vaccine, for example, the doctor includes the rubric "after vaccination" in the homeopathic workup. If the homeopath suspects the itching was triggered by an adverse reaction to a drug, the doctor would use the rubric "toxicity from drugs." Treatment is highly specific. Ten itchy animals could be prescribed ten different remedies.

Homeopaths are bombarded with difficult, seemingly hopeless cases, Richard warned as the conference concluded. Pet owners tend to seek out homeopaths only when all else failed. He even had an acronym for this—TEETH: Tried everything else, try homeopathy.

Was I up for being the vet for lost causes? I didn't know. But I was willing to try.

Chapter 40

From God's Mouth

First, I'd need to find a surgeon for Annie's compromised knee. The thicker gauge wire from surgery number three hadn't held either. I'd exhausted the best orthopedic specialists in Connecticut, so I expanded my search. I'd heard about Dr. Jerry Taylor, who'd been head orthopedic surgeon at New York City's famed Animal Medical Center for ten years. He'd opened his own hospital in Westchester, to rave reviews. And his wife was a hands-on healer!

I felt cautiously optimistic as I waited in the exam room. Annie had been through so much, including three years of failed surgeries. Taylor seemed like my last hope.

He introduced himself with a genuine smile and a warm handshake. I liked him immediately.

"Tell me what's going on with Annie."

I started at the beginning. I told him that three years earlier Annie had a partially torn ACL, and I decided to try acupuncture instead of surgery.

His eyes lit up. "Who did you go to?"

"Paul Hoffman."

"He's a friend of mine," he said. "I've referred lots of dogs to him."

I smiled. I *knew* we'd be on the same team. He *had* to be open-minded if his wife was an energy healer! "Unfortunately, it didn't help."

"Acupuncture can work wonders," he said, "but sometimes you need surgery."

I agreed. I described each of Annie's surgeries, named the surgeons, the methods used, and how they'd failed. My biggest concern, I said, was that Annie's right leg muscles were so atrophied, that I feared she'd never use her leg properly again.

Dr. Jerry listened intently. He said he wasn't surprised those methods had failed. "The only fail-safe way to fix a ruptured cruciate, is with a TPLO."

He described the Tibial Plate Leveling Osteotomy procedure in detail, but all I understood was that it involved cutting bones and inserting metal plates and screws. It sounded scary but I felt Annie was in good hands. Before returning to the receptionist to book the surgery, I asked the doctor about his wife.

"She's a graduate from the Barbara Brennan School of Healing," he told me. "You should get Barbara's book, *Hands of Light*." Barbara was a brilliant person with a degree in physics who had worked for NASA, he said.

Finally, a doctor who understood that hands-on-healing wasn't woo woo; it was actually quantum physics.

When I returned the next morning to drop Annie off for surgery, the receptionist said that Dr. Jerry had put Annie first on his list. "This way, you don't have to leave her here overnight." What a relief! Another vet who trusted my veterinary skills.

To pass the time, I drove to a nearby park where I watched the ducks for a while, tried reading in my car, and then stopped at a pizza joint for lunch. At 2 p.m. sharp, I drove back to the hospital.

The receptionist sent me straight to an exam room. Dr. Jerry entered, smiling. "Everything went well. The metal plate and screws should stabilize that knee once and for all." He advised me to limit Annie to short, slow walks and told me to bring her back in two weeks for suture removal.

Relieved, I slow-walked Annie, along with a tech, to my car, where together, we lifted her into the back seat. She slept on the hour-drive home.

I was concerned about leaving Annie alone while I worked the next day, so I arranged for my dog-sitter to check on her every few hours. When I returned from work, Annie did not look good. She was hiding under the futon and came out only after much coaxing. I managed to hand-feed her a little cooked chicken, but beyond that, she wouldn't eat. More worrisome, dark blood had seeped through the bandage.

I brought her back to Dr. Jerry the next morning for an emergency recheck.

"What's going on?" he said.

I showed him the bloodied bandage.

He cut off the dressing and inspected the incision. He told me it wasn't infected, and that sometimes surgical cuts can bleed.

He wrapped her leg with a thicker bandage, covering it with bright blue vet wrap (an elastic stretchy gauze), which applied pressure to stop the bleeding. He told me to bring her back in a few days for a bandage change.

The next morning, I noticed blood had seeped through the vet wrap. I returned to Westchester. Dr. Jerry frowned as he looked at the ugly black and blue spots on her shaved chicken leg and the dark blood leaking from the incision. He re-bandaged her and told me to come back the following day for another recheck. Next day—same thing—the blood continued to seep. I returned every day for a week. At the seventh visit, Dr. Jerry admitted he had no idea why she wasn't healing. He told me to consider euthanasia.

Put my Annie to sleep? She was only six years old! I thought I would throw up.

I cried the entire drive home.

As soon as I unleashed Annie, she crawled back under the futon. I gazed at her, my heart bursting with love. Annie was my rock. I could depend on her 100 percent. With my grandmother gone, she was the only being in the world that loved me unconditionally and who I could love back, without fear of rejection. Although I'd often wished I could provide a more spacious house and yard for my darling, mansions and money meant nothing to Annie. She'd race to follow me out the door of every friend's estate.

Annie lived for me and I for her. I couldn't let her die! I shook my head to clear my grief-fogged state. Enough of relying on even the top experts.

It was up to me. *I* had to make her better.

I looked around my living room filled with all things Annie: her tennis balls, her rawhide bones and pig ears, the green L.L. Bean flannel sheets on the chairs and sofa (those muddy feet!), the dirt-stained carpet holding memories of our daily walks at the park. Annie was the glue that held my life together. Rosemary called Annie my mother. I called her my heart.

Arnica.

The word popped into my head as if God was speaking to me. *Arnica* was the very first remedy we'd learned about at Richard's course. I ran to my office and grabbed the *Materia Medica*, a thick book filled with thousands of homeopathic remedies, along with the symptoms those remedies could cure. I needed to match the symptoms that Annie showed with the symptoms of a remedy in the book—the practical application of homeopathy's "Law of Similars."

I scanned the tiny print, single-spaced, eight pages about *Arnica*, searching for clues. I grabbed a blue pen and six-inch plastic ruler and carefully read each word, underlining everything that seemed to fit: *After surgical operations.* Annie just had knee surgery. *Septic conditions.* I hoped Annie was not septic yet. *Affects the venous system inducing stasis.* That's why the leaking blood was dark. *Black and blue spots.* All those bruises on her shaved leg. *Tendency to hemorrhage and tissue degeneration.* That's certainly what I saw. *Bruised soreness all over. Fears touch or approach of anyone. Wants to be left alone.* So that's why Annie hid under the futon. *A muscular tonic.* That's exactly what Annie needed for her thigh muscles!

This was *exactly, exactly*, what Annie displayed.

I raced upstairs to my new Professional Homeopathic Veterinary Kit that I'd purchased at the conference and selected the vial of *Arnica* 30C. I poured some tiny white granules into the cap, crouched near Annie's head, lifted her lip, and dribbled it onto her gums.

Within minutes (minutes!), her eyes brightened. She crawled out from her hiding spot, looked around the room, and spotted her Frisbee—the one that had lain unused in her toy basket for months. She grabbed it and jumped on the couch.

She jumped on the couch!

Not five minutes had passed. I couldn't believe my eyes. This must be what Richard had referred to as the *"Arnica* experience."

The next morning I un-bandaged her leg to check the incision. The bleeding had stopped and the black and blue ecchymoses had faded! She wolfed down her breakfast, her first meal in days. What a relief. That evening, twenty-four hours post-*Arnica*, her leg muscles returned. No more chicken leg—the right leg was identical to the left. This was crazy! If I hadn't seen it with my own eyes, I wouldn't have believed it. Homeopathy seemed even more miraculous than acupuncture. It seemed my Annie would be fine! Gratitude flooded through me. I called the doctor, took out the sutures myself, and never went back.

Chapter 41

A Deadly Prognosis

How could it be that this remedy, derived from a plant in the sunflower family, could prove so powerful, when other veterinary protocols had failed? Its success infused me with hope, to replicate Annie's miracles in my patients.

I didn't have long to wait. Barbara, whose German Shepherd, Duke, I'd treated successfully for arthritis, called to ask if I could help her daughter's puppy. Lexie was exhibiting some strange symptoms that her regular vet couldn't resolve.

The daughter, Melissa, arrived at my home office toting the gangly shepherd pup and the sheaf of doctor's notes I'd requested. While Lexie chewed on a rawhide bone, I focused on Melissa's story.

Melissa had brought the puppy to her local vet for a right-sided ear infection. The doctor had sold her a topical antibiotic to squirt into the dog's ear twice a day for ten days. As soon as the infection cleared up in the right ear, it appeared in the left. Melissa took the dog back to the vet. This time, he told her to put the antibiotic in both ears. She did as she was told.

The dog went deaf.

The vet referred her to a neurologist. As Melissa pondered her next step, the dog's hearing returned, along with the original right-sided ear infection. That's when Barbara told her daughter to bring the dog to me.

As Melissa explained the sequence of symptoms, I realized this was a crystal-clear example of *palliation* and *suppression*, which we'd learned about at the first homeopathic module.

Melissa's vet had *palliated* the ear infection with the first course of antibiotics, which shifted the same symptom to the other ear. Then he *suppressed* the ear infection with the second course, which cleared the body of the ear infection but drove the diseased state deeper into the body in the form of deafness. The dog's immune system did its job and fought off the deeper disease state and returned the dog to her original symptom, the right-sided ear infection.

But why did the dog have the ear infection in the first place? I had my suspicions. Discharges are the way the body tries to heal itself from toxins. (For example, we animals get diarrhea after eating bad food.) After Aspen, I was beginning to observe a pattern: that ear infections often followed a vaccine (a toxin). I studied Lexie's records. A week prior to the first ear infection, Lexie had received her DHPP puppy vaccine.

As perplexing as Lexie's condition might have appeared to her vet, this was actually quite simple. Thanks to Richard, I now knew there were several specific anti-vaccine remedies. I sent Melissa home with *Sulphur*, useful for both the bad effects of vaccines as well as suppression of discharges. A week or so later, Melissa called to tell me that Lexie's infection was gone.

I thought her vet, someone I knew and respected, would be interested in what I'd learned, so I stopped by his hospital. When I told Dr. P. that Lexie's DHPP vaccine may have triggered her ear infection, the doctor sneered: "Yeah, I pour yeast into their ears, so they have to come back for a recheck."

There was no point fighting. I thanked him for his time and left.

Meanwhile, in West Haven, Carlos, one of the techs, asked if acupuncture might help his elderly tabby's chronic constipation. Carlos, a bulldog of a guy who'd previously worked as a bouncer, said that after years of laxatives, enemas, and an occasional roto-rootering with a steel prong under anesthesia, Tony the tabby hadn't passed stool in over a week. Dr. Young told him that the next step was to remove most of the cat's colon.

We agreed to give acupuncture a try.

Although Carlos usually man-handled animals into submission, his massive hands daintily restrained his cat for me during lunch break. I'd only managed to insert a couple of needles between the dewclaws and second toes of the front legs, and two more in the rear legs before the hissing and growling began. I took the hint and stopped.

"Is that it?" Carlos asked, puzzled.

I nodded and mentally crossed my fingers, hoping four needles would suffice.

Tony tolerated the needles for five minutes. I cut my already abbreviated treatment short.

The following week, I asked about Tony. Carlos was furious. He grimaced and made farting noises with his mouth, providing a soundtrack to how his cat had squirted diarrhea all over him and his wife in their bed that night.

My treatment had worked!

The next morning, Carlos asked Dr. Young for an anti-diarrhea medication and scheduled surgery to remove the cat's colon.

A few days later, at Dr. Hunter's place in Fairfield, a woman showed up with a hairless, stinking Shar Pei. The much-coveted, excess wrinkles of this breed are caused by a genetic mutation that predisposes them to all kinds of skin disease. The skin folds around their eyes can impede vision and often necessitate surgery. These dogs are prone to thyroid disease, fungal and bacterial infections, skin irritations, folliculitis, allergies, and skin tumors. (I remember one dermatology lecture where the doctor/presenter suggested gifting our best clients Shar Peis for Christmas to ensure a steady stream of business.)

On top of that, they have nasty dispositions. Many vets, including me, wonder why people even want them.

I reviewed the dog's record. Sheba was on thyroid supplementation, prednisone, and at least two antibiotics. Her foul odor permeated the room. The miserable-looking, bald dog growled as I approached. I backed off and told Mrs. B. that I'd just returned from a holistic course where I learned that raw-meat-based diets could improve skin conditions. I handed her a photocopy of the diets that Dr. Pitcairn had created and reviewed the ingredients with her. I told her I had no idea if it would work.

"I'm desperate," she said. "I'll try anything." She left and took the Shar Pei with her.

Sheba's odor lingered behind. Fast forward six weeks. Mrs. B. returned with Sheba, paying for an office visit, just to show me the improvement made by the dog's diet: velvet-like fur covered the dog's body.

So that's what a Shar Pei should look like!

One Wednesday, a family of four, the perfect picture of poor health, entered my exam room in West Haven. They had scheduled an appointment for their allergic cat's monthly, long-acting steroid shot. I pounced. I hoped the cat could avoid those powerful steroids altogether. I put their domestic short-haired cat on the scale: twenty-four pounds, versus the ten pounds that was ideal for his frame.

"What do you feed Leo?" I said.

"Whatever dry food is on sale at the supermarket."

I explained that cats should eat a raw-meat-based diet, or at least a premium canned cat food with human-grade ingredients. "You're feeding your cat the feline equivalent of McDonald's," I said.

"What's the matter with McDonald's?" the guy snapped. "I manage a McDonalds."

I moved on. "I have a wonderful holistic product for itching," I told him. "It's a powder you add to the cat's food. It contains Biotin, a type of vitamin B."

Ignoring his sour face, I sent him home with a jar of Itch-X and an E-collar to put around the cat's neck to prevent him from licking his fur off.

Dr. Young called me later that day. He said that the owner had called, irate that I hadn't given their cat the shot. He told me I'd better stick to protocol if I wanted to keep my job.

One evening, I met a new client after hours at Dr. Hunter's place. Brian had left a message on my answering machine at home earlier that day. When I called him during my lunch break, Brian begged me to see his dog as soon as possible. He said that a board-certified internist had told him that Chloe, his seven-year old chocolate Lab, had no more than twenty-eight days to live. I agreed to see him at six o'clock.

As soon as I saw Chloe, I feared the internist had been overly optimistic. The emaciated dog could barely stand. Her head drooped and thick saliva dripped from her mouth. I could not imagine the dog would even survive a week.

While I attempted to collect myself, I lay a thick blanket on the cold tile floor in the treatment room for the dying dog. What was I getting myself into?

"Where did you get my name from?" I asked Brian.

He told me a friend had stumbled on a newspaper article about holistic veterinary medicine and after some research had found my name and number. "I can't give up on her," he said, his eyes filling with tears.

"When did this start?"

"About a month ago, Chloe began vomiting everything she ate," he said, settling down on the blanket next to his dog. "I took her to my regular vet. He took blood and told me she was in kidney failure. He said the values were off the charts and referred me to a specialist." Brian struggled to hold back his tears.

I rifled through the stack of notes that Brian handed me, searching for clues. I noticed that Chloe had received a Lyme vaccine shortly before her symptoms began. Yet the doctor maintained now that Chloe had contracted Lyme disease, which had traveled to her kidneys, shutting them down.

I looked at her bloodwork—the BUN (blood urea nitrogen) was one hundred fifty and creatinine was over twelve: the worst kidney values I had ever seen, more than six times higher than normal. When numbers are even a tad above normal, only 25 percent of the kidneys are functioning. I studied the ultrasound report. Most of Chloe's kidney tissue was necrotic, meaning dead.

Poor Chloe. We definitely needed a miracle. I remembered Simon, the old setter mix that had been resurrected, and reminded myself that no hope is false.

I kneeled on the floor next to Chloe and began a thorough physical exam. Her gums were almost white—an indication of severe anemia caused by kidney disease. All four of her legs were swollen from edema, and though she was skin and bones, her abdomen was distended— like those starving Biafran kids I'd seen in photographs. I'd never seen such an advanced state of kidney failure.

While I contemplated my next move, Brian gave me two conditions. "If Chloe is not better by tomorrow morning, I'm going to have Dr. S put in a stomach tube. He told me that's the only way to save her."

What good would force feeding her do? Certainly not heal her kidneys.

Then came the second condition. "I want you and Dr. S to work together as a team." This specialist worked alongside the guy who had called me a quack for treating IBD with acupuncture. He insisted I call the internist then and there.

Bracing myself, I dialed the hospital and got connected to Chloe's doctor. I told him in my most friendly voice that we had a mutual client at my office at the moment. "I'm a holistic vet," I explained. "Brian wants to try some alternative treatments." I felt a hostile silence but pushed on. In the spirit of camaraderie, I said, "What do you think Chloe has?"

"Autoimmune kidney disease," he grunted.

So, either the vaccine didn't work or—more likely, given the timeline—had actually caused the auto-immune disease.

"What's your prognosis?" I asked.

"She's going to die."

"In that case, would you mind if I stopped her medications?" Chloe was on heart drugs, blood pressure medications, diuretics, and antibiotics. "They will interfere with my treatment," I explained.

"Do whatever you want; the dog is going to die," my colleague stated.

So much for collaboration. Now I had to deal with the twelve-hour deadline.

Homeopathy can be somewhat of a trial and error process, so I decided to start with an acupuncture treatment, along with moxibustion, meaning the burning of a Chinese herb over the acupuncture points. After inserting needles in her kidney points, I lit the compressed cigar- shaped Chinese herb *Artemesia Vulgaris* and held the burning end over the needles for twenty minutes. After emphasizing the seriousness of her condition, I sent Brian home with a bottle of liquefied *Nux vomica*, a remedy used for the toxemia of kidney failure. I told him to call me in the morning.

And he did call me. Exuberant! Chloe was perkier and, miracle of miracles, had even eaten a full meal. No stomach tube necessary. Hurray!

Over the next few weeks, using the *Nux vomica*, followed by another homeopathic remedy, *Phosphorus*, Chloe's symptoms actually resolved—the anemia, the nausea, and the edema. She regained the twenty-five pounds she had lost and looked as good as new.

Brian decided to take her back to the specialist to show her off and repeat the bloodwork.

Brian called me after his appointment, surprised and confused. He told me that instead of being pleased with Chloe's condition, the vet was angry. He told Brian that a new experimental treatment for kidney failure using high doses of prednisone would have served Chloe better than working with a holistic vet.

Brian said he was stunned that the vet had not recommended this earlier.

I was stunned that the vet didn't acknowledge Chloe's miraculous recovery.

When Chloe's bloodwork came back from the lab the next day, Brian hand-delivered me a copy. Totally normal!

Chloe thrived for the next eighteen months. Then Brian brought her to me for a new problem. An eyelid tumor had popped up on Chloe's inner lid, causing her much discomfort. She constantly squinted and rubbed it with her paw.

This could be a problem. The anesthesia necessary for the surgical removal of the tumor could tax, probably beyond repair, Chloe's diseased kidneys. On the basis of her perfect bloodwork, Brian, as well as the surgeon, believed her kidneys were just fine. But I knew otherwise. Homeopathy can revive inflamed, dying tissue, maximizing the function of whatever viable tissue was left, but it cannot bring dead kidney tissue back to life.

Given Chloe's distress, I had to concur that, come what may, the surgery had to take place.

The dog made it through the surgery itself, but immediately afterward slid into an irreversible decline. She died four months later. Brian was heartbroken but thanked me for adding almost two years to Chloe's life. A lot more time than the four weeks the specialist had predicted.

Chapter 42

A String of Successes

One day, one of my favorite house call clients phoned for an appointment for her four young indoor cats' yearly check-ups and vaccines. And yet. At what cost to the cats? I did a quick calculation—$700 for the house call, exams, and vaccinations. My house call business was thriving. Three or four of them a month could pay my mortgage and utilities. But with all that I'd learned about vaccines, and was witnessing in my practice, I felt like a fraud. I couldn't bring myself to set up the shots. Instead, I asked how her cats were doing.

"They're wonderful!" she said.

My conscience fueled my response. "Cats don't need yearly vaccines," I told her, each word carrying a chunk of my mortgage payments.

At my conventional jobs, it seemed that all I did was vaccinate and dispense drugs. With my new knowledge, I felt I was doing my patients more harm than good. Although I'd accumulated and shared a mountain of evidence, my bosses refused to acknowledge the possibility of injury from the vaccines and drugs that we so easily administered and dispensed. At work, I felt like a walking contradiction. I found it increasingly difficult to work within these confines. Alan, my old boss, had been right after all: my philosophy and approach to medicine diverged from the mainstream.

I shared with my mother what I'd learned and what I was seeing firsthand. She shook her head at my bosses' responses. "Are they greedy? Or are they stupid?" she said.

"A little of both, I guess."

Wasn't I doing the same thing, though?

The next day, I quit my job in Oxford. I held onto my two other "day" jobs and hoped for the best.

Soon after, I was picking up my paycheck at Dr. Hunter's, when a woman returned with her eight-week-old puppy. The poor creature had stomach bloat, a potentially life-threatening condition that typically affects big-chested adult dogs, like Great Danes. I'd never seen a puppy with bloat. According to the owner, the little guy had bloated within an hour of his DHPP vaccine.

I overheard my boss tell the owner that the bloat had been caused by something the dog ate. Yet the owner insisted the dog hadn't eaten anything that day. The doctor gave the dog a shot of antibiotics and dispensed an antacid to be taken daily. After the owner left, I questioned Dr. Hunter about this. "The bloat occurred an hour after the shot. How could this not be related?" I asked. He mumbled something and turned away.

The very next week, a woman dropped off her fifteen-year-old black Lab for a flea and tick bath and dip, as well as its vaccines. This dog was in "uncompensated heart failure," Dr. Hunter had written in the dog's thick record. This meant that despite a slew of heart meds, the dog's heart was not functioning, and the animal was in all probability close to death.

Vaccine inserts state that vaccinations are for "healthy animals only." Could anyone call this old Labrador healthy? Absolutely not. I muttered to Darlene, the receptionist, that I couldn't vaccinate this sick dog. In my heart, I couldn't rationalize it.

A few minutes later, Darlene called me to the phone. Dr. Hunter was on the line, and he was furious. "Darlene told me you won't vaccinate that dog. Any dog that is not dying on the table gets all of its vaccines!"

It seemed as if I'd been ordered to kill this dog; Darlene stood sentry, making sure that I carried out the boss's dictates. I felt sick as I injected him.

When I returned home that night, I couldn't get that old black Lab out of my mind. Vaccinating him was counter to everything I'd learned and what I knew to be true. I handed in my notice on my next day there.

This left my West Haven job, the least challenging to my integrity. Most patients that came through that door were ill and needed help. Only rarely did animals come for yearly boosters. I needed this last steady paycheck. I tried to convince myself that keeping this job was okay.

I could now devote six free days a week to my growing holistic practice. The newspaper articles and my TV appearance continued to generate a steady stream of clients. I called my business the Animal Natural Healing Center and printed some business cards.

I could also devote more time to my pro bono work. Bill, a volunteer from New Leash on Life, called one day to set up an appointment for a corgi-mix he was fostering.

"Lucas can barely walk. He's already been to three veterinarians, including a specialist," Bill said. The treatments from all three vets not only didn't help, but they had made Lucas sicker, according to Bill. "You are our last hope." I'd heard this from clients more than once. Many people, it seemed, reached out to me when conventional medicine had failed.

I requested the doctors' notes, including X-rays, from all three vets and asked Bill to bring them and Lucas to my home office later that week.

Bill arrived carrying the forty-plus-pound dog and placed him on a comforter on my wood floor. Bill handed me the pile of notes and two big manila envelopes filled with X-rays, then sat on the floor next to Lucas.

I pulled out a fresh treatment record. "Please start from the beginning."

"When we got Lucas from the shelter, he refused to walk," Bill said. "We brought him to our local vet, who took an X-ray. He said Lucas had a broken back and had probably been hit by a car. The vet gave him some drugs for pain, but the pills gave Lucas terrible diarrhea, and he still couldn't walk."

I glanced down at Lucas, his head trembling on Bill's leg.

Bill opted for a second opinion from his friend's vet. That vet took more X-rays and told Bill that Lucas had an enlarged heart and was in heart failure. This doctor prescribed powerful cardiac drugs and diuretics, which made Lucas vomit. The dog grew weaker and still couldn't walk.

At a loss, Bill decided to confer with a specialist. Nearly a thousand dollars spent on tests later, the board-certified internist told Bill that Lucas had Cushing's disease. He started the dog on chemotherapy, which, Bill said, nearly killed the dog. That's when Bill remembered me. He hadn't thought of holistic treatment, but with nowhere else to turn, he decided to call.

I asked Bill to lift the dog onto the exam table. Lucas smiled up at me, and I smiled back. What a strange looking creature! Mostly corgi, he had a large, long body, low to the ground, with a big head and ears, disproportionate to the rest of him.

I began a thorough physical exam. First, I looked in his mouth. I couldn't believe my eyes: judging by his teeth, I gauged that Lucas could be no more than nine months old. He was still a puppy! I looked in his eyes with my ophthalmoscope, checked his ears with my otoscope: all normal. I listened carefully to his heart with my stethoscope, checking for a murmur, which could indicate a compromised heart. Completely normal.

As I worked my way down his body, I stopped short: Lucas had no front legs! Well, not none, exactly: like the Thalidomide children—thousands born with severe birth defects after their mothers took an anti-morning-sickness drug—he had no arms, just paws attached to his trunk, like flippers. An apparent congenital deformity. This was why Lucas couldn't walk: He had no front legs!

Three vets supposedly examined him and didn't note that he had no front legs?

Still, I didn't say anything until I reviewed the test results.

Since I didn't have an X-ray viewer, I held up the X-rays one by one to the spotlight on my ceiling. My jaw dropped. Lucas' entire spine was filled with arthritis. I'd never seen this in a puppy.

The only logical explanation was that the steep tilt of Lucas' back had put undue pressure on his spine, causing the arthritis. (I could sort of understand why the first vet had thought the dog had been hit by a car.) Lucas groaned and winced as I pressed gently along each and every intervertebral space. Poor little guy.

Next, I removed the chest X-ray from the second manila envelope and held that up to the light, searching for any sign of heart failure. There was no fluid in the lungs, but the heart did appear to be slightly bigger than I'd expect for a dog this size. But given that Lucas was a corgi-mix, I felt it totally appropriate. I'd learned from Alan that dwarf-type dogs, like basset hounds, dachshunds, and corgis, often have a disproportionate heart-to-chest-size ratio.

Next I turned to the blood tests, looking for abnormalities. Yes, the alkaline phosphatase, an enzyme that can be of either bone or liver origin, was somewhat elevated. But in a puppy, this elevation is totally normal and due to rapidly growing bones. It's not an indication of disease. The level of the enzyme was nowhere near what an older dog with Cushing's disease would have, where the liver would be hyper-secreting the enzyme.

I shook my head in disbelief at these misdiagnoses. How could three vets with much more experience than I get it so wrong? Had anyone actually *examined* the dog?

"Your dog has no front legs."

Bill's eyes widened. "The groomer told me there was something wrong with his legs!"

"Look."

Lucas's body was so close to the ground and he was so hairy that if you didn't look closely you wouldn't notice it. But groomers would. They go over the dogs with a fine-tooth comb, literally and figuratively.

After three pro bono acupuncture treatments, Lucas moved well enough to join Bill and his wife on walks with their other two rescues. The couple decided to adopt him.

Steve and Tiffany, recent transplants from Manhattan, brought their Akita, Tasha, to my home office one day. They arrived with a huge rolling suitcase filled with doctors' notes. I'd become accustomed to hundreds of pages of vets' records, but this suitcase business was a first.

Tasha had been diagnosed with immune-mediated polyarthritis, a condition common to Akitas. (Though conventional medicine labeled this disease as having no recognized cause, I immediately thought *vaccine-injury*, per my recent studies.)

Steve told me that the Animal Medical Center had used Tasha as a case study. Ruffling through the mountain of papers, I had to ask how much the couple had spent on their dog's care. "Let's put it this way," Steve said dryly, "we could have bought a Porsche." I hadn't a clue what a Porsche cost, but I imagined, a lot. Despite this outlay for whatever diagnoses and treatments, Tasha could barely walk because of the pain.

I decided to start with acupuncture, as it can give immediate relief. However, inserting needles into painful joints can sometimes hurt. I noticed that Tasha, like most Akitas, had a challenging temperament (to put it mildly), so I told Tiffany to feed Tasha treats, while Steve restrained her. Tasha didn't fall for it. When her warning growls turned serious, I had to use a muzzle, a rarity in my office.

After ten weekly sessions, which cost less than a good bicycle, Tasha was pain-free.

A few months after Tasha, I met a dying six-year-old Shetland sheepdog named Bella. The specialist at the veterinary referral hospital had diagnosed Bella with acute kidney failure. When Ellen, the owner, called me about a potential appointment, she told me that Bella hadn't responded to the specialist's treatment of aggressive IV fluid therapy and lots of drugs. After three days in the hospital, Bella still wouldn't eat and continued to vomit. And the dog's bloodwork hadn't improved one iota. The vets had told Ellen that the only option was euthanasia. Ellen, a dentist, had refused their recommendation and sought my help.

I settled the exhausted and frail sheltie on a blanket on my office floor. Daunted by the thick manila envelope filled with doctors' notes, I turned to Ellen and asked what had happened.

Her story poured out: Bella had never had a single medical problem until a few days prior. Ellen had applied a new flea and tick product between the dog's shoulder blades. One hour after the application, Bella began to vomit bile and then guzzle water, only to vomit that up as well. She rushed the dog to the emergency hospital.

"I told them just what I told you," the young dentist said with obvious frustration. She figured it was the liquid insecticide that she'd bought from the vet. "They said it was impossible for the tick stuff to cause kidney failure, because it's not absorbed into the blood." The vet insisted that, according to the product insert, the poison stays in the sebaceous glands.

But Ellen suspected otherwise. As a medical practitioner, she knew there could be unexpected side effects to drugs. She emphasized that the dog had been totally healthy prior to the flea/tick medication, but the vets dismissed her conclusion and ran a battery of every test available (including for Rocky Mountain Spotted Fever, the incidence of which in Connecticut was exactly zero). After thousands of dollars of testing, the doctors still hadn't come up with an explanation for why the dog was dying.

There's a saying in medicine: "When you hear hoofbeats, think of horses, not zebras." Meaning look for the most obvious things first.

I turned to the pile of records and headed straight for the renal ultrasound report. It stated that Bella's kidneys were *hypoplastic*, meaning she had been born with abnormally small kidneys, a condition I'd seen before in shelties. She must have absorbed the medicine into her bloodstream and filtered it through her defective kidneys. Most likely, her already weak kidneys were unable to eliminate and detoxify the poisonous insecticide.

We had no time to waste—the dog was at death's door. I started her on a low daily dose of *Nux vomica*, the homeopathic remedy I was turning to again and again to help pets poisoned by drugs. I added a couple of herbal supplements to support the kidneys.

The very next morning, Ellen reported that Bella was brighter, had stopped vomiting, and had even eaten some chicken baby food.

Chapter 43

A Death and Resurrection

Emboldened by my successes, I leapt off the cliff and quit my remaining day job in West Haven.

Brenda called soon after about her shepherd, Max. I'd been treating Max's elbow dysplasia since I'd started acupuncture and had treated him the previous week, so her call surprised me. Apparently, Max was limping badly on his right front leg. I told her to bring Max over immediately.

I watched Max walk—the limp *was* pronounced—then Brenda restrained him while I examined the leg. Max cried out when I palpated his carpus (wrist). His other joints showed no pain. I gave him an acupuncture treatment for wrist pain, and drew blood to send to the lab to check for Lyme disease. "Call me in two days," I told her, since I was going out of town for a couple of days and the bloodwork would be in by the time I got back.

When I checked my phone messages the next day, Brenda was desperate. I called her back. Max was worse, so I told her to take him to Jerry Taylor, the orthopedic vet, for an X-ray. I gave her Jerry's number and told her to have the hospital fax me the report.

Early the next morning, before I'd even had a chance to check my faxes, Brenda called. "Max has bone cancer," she said between sobs. "I called my mother. She's flying in from Texas to be with me when I put him to sleep."

"What?" I shouted into the phone. "Hold on a second."

I ran to my fax machine. Dr. Jerry had X-rayed Max and diagnosed osteosarcoma (bone cancer) of the elbow. I rushed back to the phone.

"Taylor told me he needs to amputate Max's leg, otherwise I should put him to sleep," Brenda sobbed. "He's ten years old with arthritis. I can't cut his leg off—I love him too much."

"Bring Max right over," I told Brenda. "I want to have a look at him."

Half an hour later, my tearful friend perched anxiously on my living room sofa while I sat cross-legged on the carpet with Max. How could this dog have had only a painful carpus two days ago and now have bone cancer of his elbow? This didn't make sense.

I lifted the bad leg and began a methodical exam, starting at the toes. Pus oozed from one of the nail beds. I hadn't noticed that before. I checked the other toes; they were fine. I palpated his carpus—no pain. That was odd; he'd cried out just a couple of days prior. I manipulated his elbow—mild pain, but nothing more than I'd expect with arthritis. When I tried to flex and extend his shoulder, Max screamed.

How strange. Taylor said that Max had cancer of his elbow, not his shoulder. I knew it could be difficult to distinguish severe osteoarthritis from cancer on an X-ray, but this didn't add up. Plus, the pus was a red flag.

I remembered reading about ascending infections in vet school in Italy. These infections could start from a wound and travel upward. *As in starting in a nail bed and migrating up to the shoulder?* An ascending infection was the only thing that made sense to me. Max had a painful wrist on Sunday, a painful elbow on Monday, and a painful shoulder on Tuesday. I suspected that Max had injured his nail and the infection had progressed upward from there.

I didn't think he had bone cancer. Were amputation or euthanasia the only choices for this shepherd? I didn't think so.

I knew that the homeopathic remedy *Silicea* could be useful for infections of the nail bed. I grabbed my *Materia Medica* and looked up the symptoms—an ascending infection, the pus, the pain. I prepared a bottle of the remedy and told Brenda to give it to Max twice daily.

When Brenda left, I called Dr. Jerry and told him about the nail bed infection and the painful shoulder. "It *has* to be an ascending infection," I insisted.

He seemed doubtful. "I learned about them in vet school," he said, "but in thirty years of practice, I've never seen a case."

"Me either," I agreed. "But I think we have one here."

Two days later Brenda called. Max was much better. The pus had dried up, and his limp had improved. Brenda's mother cancelled her flight.

(Max lived many years more.)

A parade of clients came to me with dying animals. I felt like Humpty-Dumpty, picking up the pieces of broken animals and trying to put them together again. Sometimes, I felt like Sisyphus, the guy from the Greek myth condemned to repeatedly roll that boulder up a hill, only to have it tumble down again.

A year and a half after I treated Tasha (that temperamental Akita who generated a Porsche-worth of vet payments), Steve called again. "Tasha can't walk," he said.

"What happened?"

"I don't know. She's been great, but all of a sudden she can't get up."

Something must have caused her to crash. "Did you give her any vaccines?"

"Nooooo," Steve said. "We brought her to the regular vet two days ago. We told them no vaccines—they only did a heartworm test. But," he paused, "they put some new flea and tick stuff between her shoulders. Do you think that could have caused this?"

Oy vey.

I recommended he bring his dog to my office, but after a discussion with his wife, they decided to euthanize Tasha. They couldn't bear to see her suffer anymore.

All this suffering by these poor creatures and so much of it unnecessary.

Then a dog died under my care. But only temporarily.

Annette, a volunteer I knew from New Leash on Life, asked if I would cut her Dobie's nails. Lady wouldn't let Annette do it. She would become frantic, fight, and even bite, like many dogs do. Of course, I'd do it.

Annette had a regular vet, so I didn't bother to examine the dog; this was just a pedicure, after all. I started with Lady's rear paws, as most dogs tolerate those better. By the time I reached for a front leg though, Lady panicked. She struggled and then went limp and collapsed. I glanced at the dog's face—the pupils were dilated. I lifted a lip—the gums were blue. A pool of urine had leaked onto the floor.

Lady was dead.

"Annette, your dog just died," I squeaked.

I grabbed the fifty-remedy emergency kit I kept on my bookshelf. Hand shaking, Eustachian tube collapsing, I managed to pull out a vial of *Carbo veg*, which Dr. Pitcairn had called the "corpse reviver." I poured some pellets straight from the bottle onto Lady's blue gums.

The dog popped up, seemingly good as new.

"She's back," I croaked.

Annette looked confused. The fact that her dog had died and come back to life hadn't registered.

I grabbed my stethoscope and listened to the dog's heart. I detected a significant heart murmur. Doberman Pinschers are prone to dilated cardio-myopathy. This progressive and fatal heart condition can cause arrhythmias (irregular heartbeats) that lead to sudden death.

"Annette," I said, "do you know your dog has a bad heart murmur?"

Annette, still in a state of shock, shook her head no.

I ran upstairs to my stockroom and prepared a bottle of liquefied *Carbo veg* (multiple doses and easy to administer) for Annette to take home. "Call a cardiologist for an ultrasound as soon as possible," I told her. "In the meantime, if Lady collapses, squirt a third of the dropper straight into the dog's mouth. Call me with any updates."

The cardiologist faxed over his ultrasound a few days later, confirming my diagnosis. When I called Annette to discuss the results, she said that Lady had collapsed twice: once when she climbed onto the curb and again when she went up the stairs. Each time, the *Carbo veg* had revived the dog within seconds.

After the crush of business, the stream of phone calls slowed to a trickle.

Then nothing.

At first, I didn't mind. In fact, I rather enjoyed it. Between vet school, my grueling work schedule, and my holistic courses, I hadn't had any down time in twenty years!

I caught up on errands, cleaned the attic, purged files of papers, organized stacks of notes, and refolded my clothes neatly in their drawers. When there was nothing more to organize or clean, I even started to relax.

By the third month, though, I started getting anxious. I didn't do vaccines anymore and I'd given up my day jobs, so I wasn't earning money. I had bills to pay.

Maybe going off on my own had been a huge mistake.

One day, as I moved toward the non-blinking answering machine again, a deep voice behind me thundered: *"You take care of the ones that you have, and I will take care of the rest!"*

I turned around, even though I knew nobody was there. The voice sounded like what I imagined Moses must have heard from the burning bush.

That message was so clear, that I knew it to be *Truth*, a commandment both powerful and comforting.

God told me not to worry. I let go.

The very next day, my phone started ringing off the hook again.

Chapter 44

A Thanksgiving Miracle

Dr. David Ulrich, an eighty-year-old psychologist, was on the line. His three-year-old Golden Retriever-mix, Phoebe, had been hit by a car and was at the Darien Animal Hospital, paralyzed and in a lot of pain. The orthopedic surgeon at the hospital, my old friend Dr. McCarthy, said Phoebe would have a 10 percent chance of recovery with surgery, a full body cast, and six months of rehab. He suggested euthanasia as the kindest option, David said.

David asked the surgeon if acupuncture might help. "Dr. McCarthy said that acupuncture would be a total waste of money," David told me, "and that it couldn't help with the structural damage of the spine."

David got my name from Dr. Joseph Ho, an acupuncturist I used for my own health.

"Do you think you can help?" David asked, his voice cracking with emotion.

I felt overwhelmed by the gravity of this situation. A broken back and dissected spine sounded beyond repair. "I really don't know," I said, "but I can give you the same odds as Dr. McCarthy, without surgery and a full body cast." (And for a tiny fraction of the cost.)

I wanted to help this poor dog, but I'd need a hospital to board her, as David said he couldn't manage her at home, and I didn't have a facility. Then I remembered that Dr. Adam Butler, a colleague from Italy, owned a hospital in Stratford, about twenty-five minutes from my house. Graduates from Italian vet schools tended to be more open-minded than American-trained vets.

I called Dr. Adam and promised I'd drive to his hospital three times a week to treat the dog. Dr. Adam said he was happy to help out. I called David back with the good news.

I had no idea what to expect the next morning as I raced to Stratford, my car loaded with acupuncture needles, my electrical acupuncture stimulation device, some herbal supplements, and a handful of homeopathic remedies.

The receptionist led me to the treatment area, where Alan greeted me and led me to our patient. A beautiful golden-haired dog lay on a blanket in the middle of the room, howling in pain. Her crying sent chills up my spine.

"Can I see her radiographs?" I asked.

Dr. Adam put the X-rays in the viewer.

I gasped. The spine was dissected in half! One section of the spine sat on top of the another, like a layer cake. Now I understood why the orthopedic surgeon had said that acupuncture wouldn't work. There was 100 percent displacement of two of her vertebrae. Phoebe couldn't move her legs or her tail and couldn't urinate or defecate on her own. Her back end lay useless, like a limp rag. I had cured many cases of partial paralysis in dachshunds, but I had never seen anything like this.

From the hospital, I called David at his home in Lyme, as promised, to discuss Phoebe's condition.

David had already spoken with Dr. Adam that morning. David and his wife, Judy, had decided that if Phoebe did not improve in forty-eight hours, they would put her to sleep. They couldn't bear to leave her in such pain.

I hung up the phone, opened my backpack, took out my stuff, and set to work. I inserted the acupuncture needles, hooked them up to the electrical machine, and sat cross-legged in front of Phoebe. Gently, I took her paw, closed my eyes, and began to pray.

After the twenty-minute treatment, I showed Dr. Adam how to administer the homeopathic medicine *Hypericum*, remedy par excellence for the treatment of nerve damage. Phoebe would need it three times daily. I showed him how to prepare a castor oil pack, an old-fashioned treatment that I'd found effective for disk disease. I added a few supplements and vitamins to the regimen, but my heart felt heavy as I left the office.

I called Dr. Adam on Day Two to check in. There'd been no change. Further, when David had visited the hospital the previous evening, Phoebe had ignored him. David and his wife decided to put Phoebe to sleep the following day, so that they could be with her when Dr. Adam injected the euthanasia solution.

But in the morning of Day Three, Adam called the Ulrichs. Phoebe had stopped crying and had urinated on her own. He suggested they postpone the euthanasia, and they did as he suggested.

On Day Four, when I arrived at the hospital for the second treatment, Phoebe managed a feeble wag of her tail when she saw me. She wagged her tail! The spinal cord worked! Although Dr. Adam was thrilled with the improvement, he remained skeptical that she would ever walk again.

When I called David for our daily check-in, he told me about *his* work on Phoebe's behalf. He'd had some training in Reiki, a method of energy healing, where the practitioner puts their hands over the diseased area to send healing waves. Since he couldn't get to Phoebe in person, he'd started performing Reiki on a teddy bear, mindfully transmitting energy via the stuffed animal to his ailing dog. "Who knows?" the eighty-year-old psychologist exclaimed. "We are in the New Age after all!"

A little miracle followed each acupuncture treatment: Phoebe moved a paw, the clicking sound in her spine stopped, she was able to stand, she took a step . . .

Bolstered by her improved mental and physical state, David and Judy took Phoebe home on the day before Thanksgiving, only fourteen days after her first treatment. No surgery, no cast, no rehab.

With Grandma gone and no family around, I'd created a ritual to get me through Thanksgiving: I'd choose a film and take myself to a matinee, where I'd sit alone in the almost empty movie theatre. When I returned home from the cinema that day, I got David's message. He said that when they sat down to dinner, Phoebe heaved herself up on her forelegs and stared at them indignantly, as if to say: "How dare you start without me?" She then dragged herself over to her usual position, under the table, to take her rightful place as part of the family. Although *we* might forget how important it is to be together at mealtimes, Phoebe certainly didn't. "I think it was a canine way of saying grace," he said.

Before the hospital had discharged Phoebe, I'd shown David a rudimentary form of reflexology—a kind of deep massage between Phoebe's hind paw pads. I'd told him to do it five minutes, twice daily. David reported that on Thanksgiving morning, after her treatment, Phoebe began to scratch her ear with her paw. When David watched that leg fly back and forth, he said, he knew everything would be ok.

What a beautiful gift this was to me on Thanksgiving Day. David's message reminded me of God's plans for my life. Knowing that I'd played a part in the Ulrichs' joyful Thanksgiving reunion eased my struggles and bolstered my spirit.

David dropped Phoebe at the Stratford hospital twice weekly for my treatments, and we spoke daily. He took special delight in explaining their improvised management techniques. In order to get Phoebe up the stairs at night without hurting the dog's spine, "we all moved in sync like a six-legged creature," David enthused.

Day by day, Phoebe improved. After her twelfth acupuncture treatment (in the course of six weeks), Phoebe "ran out the door and shot like a rocket after a squirrel," David said.

He and Judy decided to take Phoebe back to Dr. McCarthy, the orthopedic vet who had told him to not waste his money on acupuncture, for a visit.

When Phoebe walked in, according to David, the surgeon said, "What is this? What did you do?" Dr. McCarthy grabbed the leash and led Phoebe into the back for a follow up X-ray, as Judy told him about the acupuncture.

When he returned, the surgeon placed Phoebe's two X-rays—the first from the time of the accident, and the second, post-treatment—side by side on the viewer. The doctor stood back and stared, shaking his head, according to David. He called in the entire staff to look at the "miracle," David said. He noted a 100 percent reduction in the displacement of the vertebrae, meaning the structural damage of the spine was completely healed. "It's enough to make you a believer. Marcie should be proud of herself!" David recalled him saying. At that moment, I felt my heart bursting with love and gratitude toward God—for gifting me the opportunity to work as His instrument in this Divine healing.

David stayed in touch. He told me that the $1200 cart that Dr. Adam had encouraged him to purchase when Phoebe couldn't walk had made a beautiful planter. David said that he and Judy kept the doggie wheelchair in the living room as a reminder of their grace.

Chapter 45

Dreams of Manhattan

In 1998, I began to have the strangest dreams. Every night, I dreamed that I moved to New York City. The dreams were filled with—there is no other word for it—bliss. "But I don't want to work in New York City," I'd say out loud as I woke up from yet another dream. Despite my resistance, it became clear that *someone* was trying to tell me something.

Unable to ignore the dreams any longer, I opened the new veterinary journal to the classified section, where an ad caught my eye. The only holistic pet store in Manhattan, Whiskers, sought a holistic vet to partner with.

A gift dropped from heaven? I had no idea. I called.

Later, as I boarded a Metro North train to New York City for the interview, I felt as if I were an actor in a play. For years I'd watch commuters rush to the train while I took Annie on her morning walk around Fairfield town center. I'd feel myself in their shoes. I somehow *knew* that I should be wearing my backpack and moving along with the rest of them.

I hadn't been to New York City since Grandma had died six years earlier. New York was Grandma, and Grandma was gone. The thought of being there without her had been too painful to bear. But when I disembarked from the train and exited the terminal, I wanted to bend down and kiss the sidewalk. Just like in my dreams!

The interview went well, but I was not quite ready to commit to a partnership. I agreed to accept referrals for house calls in New York and to move forward from there.

A couple of weeks later, I strode through the streets of Manhattan on the way to my first house call, the winter sun shining bright and warm on my head. I hadn't realized how much I missed city life. I felt I had the world at my feet. I remembered Dr. Hoffman say that some of his colleagues had begged him to work out of their offices in Manhattan, as there were no certified veterinary acupuncturists in the city. Could I be the only one?

Whiskers's referrals led to weekly commutes to New York. On Week Four, as I strode down to Greenwich Village for my second client of the day, a now familiar thrill coursed through me like a current. I rang the bell and got buzzed in. A young, petite, dark-haired woman and a sweet, fluffy, black and white dog greeted me. After the introductions, I set my computer and papers on the dining room table and we got down to business.

Tara had explained prior to our visit that Sadie, her little rescue dog, had chronic digestive problems that at least three vets hadn't helped. She handed me the doctors' notes that I'd requested. I searched for the date prior to the first episode of diarrhea. I'd discovered that most maladies began with either vaccinations, flea and tick medicines, drugs, or emotions—usually grief. I had seen time and again that when a companion animal died, an owner fell sick, or the pet's owners went on vacation, leaving their animal with a pet sitter (even the favorite one), the pet crashed! Emotions, just like vaccines and drugs, are a huge stress to the immune system and can cause a new problem or trigger a flare-up of a pet's underlying chronic disease.

Sadie had received her set of yearly boosters the day prior to the first bout of diarrhea. I included the rubric "after vaccinations" in my homeopathic workup. As I worked my way through the notes, I noticed that Sadie's diarrhea had worsened after a course of antibiotics the vet had dispensed for a cut toe pad. This indicated a drug sensitivity, as not all dogs got diarrhea from antibiotics, so I typed "oversensitive to medicines" into her chart. The medications dispensed by the vets had helped Sadie's diarrhea temporarily, only to recur shortly after the drugs were stopped. This was palliation, which I added to the mix.

I questioned Tara about all Sadie's physical symptoms—from the time she'd rescued the dog until the present. It seemed that when Tara had gone on vacation and left the dog with her boyfriend, the diarrhea had flared up. Emotional and physical sensitivity go hand-in-hand. I added "ailments from grief," another rubric I'd found helpful.

It looked like Sadie had inflammatory bowel disease. At my previous job with the partners, Alan had purchased an endoscope and had biopsied dozens and dozens of dogs with chronic diarrhea. I always kidded him: "Why do you need to do this? You always get the same results: lymphocytic-plasmacytic enteritis," otherwise known as IBD. He might have found cancer in an older dog, but in all the years I was there, he never did.

Then I took Tara through the list of questions I'd created regarding a pet's mental and emotional makeup. Tara told me that Sadie followed her from room to room in the apartment, never letting her owner out of her sight. She slept in bed with Tara, her little body pressed right up against her owner. If Tara was sad, Sadie would stick by her like glue and even lick away her tears!

It took about an hour to complete my three-page list of questions. Tara confirmed that I now knew more about her dog than Tara herself had an hour earlier.

I moved on to the physical exam. While Tara sat on the rug with Sadie, I examined the dog from head to tail. From the outside, Sadie looked terrific.

I returned to my computer, inserted a few more rubrics, and then double-checked some remedies from the *Materia Medica* that I'd lugged in my backpack. Choosing a correct homeopathic remedy, in the best-case scenario, can seem like a superhuman feat. There are over three thousand remedies. The incorrect ones will do nothing at all. Remedies that are similar, but not spot on, can temporarily aggravate symptoms. Only one or two will help, but the correct dosage is important. If it's given in too high a dose, the remedy can cause an exacerbation of one or more symptoms. Although this "healing crisis" is positive, an indication of self-healing, it can freak out the owner. On the other hand, if the remedy is administered in too low a dose, the remedy wouldn't work, and the owner may give up.

I decided that *Pulsatilla* (made from a type of windflower) fit the picture. I decided on a low daily dose and directed Tara to a local pharmacy where she could purchase it.

Tara looked dazed and awed as she watched me work. "Why don't you open an office in the Village?" she said. "There are no good vets around here. You'd have a booming business."

While I loved Greenwich Village, the cost of Manhattan real estate was way beyond my means. "I don't know how I could afford it," I found myself telling her.

Tara said, "I have a good friend who is a commercial realtor. I'm sure he can help you."

Could things move this fast? The dreams had only started two months before!

The instant I left her apartment, rain started coming down like cats and dogs, so I rushed to the corner to hail a taxi. The cabs were either filled or had their off-duty lights on. I was getting soaked and started to panic as I had all my supplies on me and remembered that it was next to impossible to get a taxi in New York in the rain. It occurred to me to pray. I'd never asked God for anything as trivial as a taxi, but I had to get home to Annie, and I didn't want to lose my gear.

Just as I said my first, "Please God," a cab with its off-duty sign lit up pulled over. What a relief! I was mystified and had to ask, "Why did you stop if you are off-duty?"

"Everyone was trying to flag me down," he said. "I didn't pick them up because I was in a hurry to get home. Something told me to stop for that woman." Meaning me.

"I was praying for a taxi," I confessed.

"I pray all the time," he said.

Who knows why I never thought taxi drivers to be the praying type. I suddenly felt a heart-to-heart connection with this guy. "What do you pray for?" I asked.

"I pray I don't hit anybody and that nobody hits me," he said.

The next morning, I called Tara's realtor friend, Ben, and introduced myself.

"Tara told me you'd call," he said. "I have a fantastic office space in the best part of the Village—on West 11th Street, just off 4th Street."

We made a date to meet the following day.

As I walked toward the address, I looked around in amazement. Despite years of living in Manhattan, I'd never known this part of the Village existed. It was so European—with its cobblestoned, tree-lined streets, quaint boutiques, and locals sitting on their stoops with their pet cats. I felt like I was in Italy or France, in the daydream of my night dream.

A slight young man in jeans and a down parka looked like he was waiting for someone. I figured it was Ben and introduced myself.

"Hi, Marcie. Tara told me all about you. She's a good friend of mine. You're in luck—this space just came on the market. I think you'll love it!"

I followed him down a narrow, open-backed metal stairwell to a basement office. Ben unlocked the door and I stepped into a newly renovated dream space. A narrow, brick-walled entry hall (*waiting room!*) led to a new, marble-floored bathroom. Ben led the way into a spacious, brick-walled room (*exam room!*) with shiny, new, wood floors. Sun streamed in the front windows. We doubled back through the entrance to a rear room (*storage room!*) which was nearly as large, its two windows opening into an alley.

I fell in love. "How much is the rent?" I questioned, expecting the worst.

"$1000 a month. You can't beat that!"

This seemed almost too good to be true. "Is this office zoned for veterinarians?" I knew that animal hospitals need special commercial zoning, but I was in a gray area, as I didn't do surgery, use or dispense drugs, perform euthanasia, or board or hospitalize animals. But I didn't want to risk any illegality.

"Well, not officially. But the landlord doesn't care," Ben reassured me. "I told him your situation."

The stairs worried me. Open-backed stairs scare dogs, particularly those with difficulty walking. My patients included many large, crippled, and paralyzed dogs. I figured most city dogs would be small, but I didn't know how I would get the bigger ones up and down those stairs.

I told Ben I had to think about it.

"Don't think too long," he told me. "This place will be snapped up."

On the train home to Fairfield, I prayed for a sign.

Chapter 46

The Right Wrong Number

When I arrived home, I took Annie for a quick walk and then checked my phone messages. A reporter from the *New York Times* had called. She wanted to interview me!

My hand shook as I dialed the number.

The reporter picked up. She was doing a story on animals and acupuncture, and she wanted to interview me in person. "Would you be available?" she said.

Would I?! "Where did you get my name from?" I asked, trying to control my excitement.

"From the American Holistic Veterinary Medical Association's list of veterinarians in New York."

I hesitated. "Do I need to have an office in New York City?"

"Absolutely," she said. "Don't you have one?"

This was the sign I'd prayed for. "Yes!"

She asked for the address, adding that she'd need a client and patient for the interview.

I had to think fast: my office space, which I hadn't yet secured, but I was already calling my own, wouldn't be ready in time. Then I thought of Phoebe, with the cured broken back, and David, the psychologist. David had a Manhattan apartment! I knew he'd be happy to help. I told Margalit, the reporter, the short version of Phoebe's broken back and how acupuncture had cured it. "Why don't we meet at my client's apartment?" I queried, trying to sound as casual as possible.

"Sounds perfect."

Phew.

We set a date and a time, and as soon as I hung up, I called Ben and told him I was ready to sign the lease. Then I called my parents to tell them the good news. The *New York Times*!

On the day of the interview, I drove into the city, a first for me. As I started to make a left-hand-turn, I found myself facing six lanes of oncoming traffic stopped at a red light. I froze. Thankfully, a cop noticed my situation and shooed me into the gas station on the corner. Somehow, I made it. Phoebe greeted me at the door with David, who led me into the living room and introduced me to Margalit and the photographer.

Before the actual interview began, I told Margalit I needed to ask her something. "Why did you choose my name from the AHVMA's list of veterinarians?"

"Actually," she said, "I meant to call Dr. Jordan, who was listed as a board-certified neurologist and acupuncturist from the Animal Medical Center, but I must have misdialed. When I heard your voice message, I realized my mistake. But I figured, what the heck, you'd be fine for the interview."

Divine intervention.

My next order of business after the interview was to actually move into my new office. I called Mom and told her that I wanted to install a Murphy bed for overnight stays, in case I worked late. Mom loved the idea. "You can have a life now! You'll finally meet other single people and go out and have some fun. I told you years ago, you belong in Manhattan."

Mom offered to meet me at the Murphy bed store in Manhattan to help choose things for the office. In addition to beds, the store built made-to-order furniture. This sounded perfect. I wanted everything to be perfect—this would be my dream office, both literally and figuratively.

Mom and I spoke briefly to the salesperson and then followed him into the rear showroom. After double-checking measurements, I chose a light pine, full-sized Murphy bed with a side hutch. The hutch had shelves and drawers and a space to hang clothes. When the bed folded down it exposed three adorable overhead night lights. It looked so cozy; I could imagine myself curling up with a good book after a day's work. With the bed raised into the storage position, it looked just like a wardrobe. No one would suspect a thing.

I decided on a large wooden bench seat, in matching pine, for the waiting room. The custom bench would seat four skinny people or three normal-sized ones, and could double as storage for my blankets and pillows. Tufted forest green pillows would add a rustic, welcoming touch, my mom said.

I unearthed my elegant Italian diploma (which had taken me ten years to earn and another ten for the University of Bologna to print) and my official New York State License (with God's grace, I'd passed the test the first time I took it) from my attic and chose some of the newspaper articles about me to frame. My handyman, Ken, rented a U-Haul van and transported me and my stuff into the City.

I unpacked the many boxes of supplements, remedies, and books, while Ken installed and assembled the air conditioning units, cabinets, bookcases, and more. I placed a sterling silver cat business-card holder on the desk and tucked inside the cards I'd designed with my new West 11th Street address. In the place of honor, centered on the red brick wall of the exam room, Ken hung a poster Colette had gifted me for my birthday: a shaggy black pony, a honey-colored Jersey cow, a fluffy collie, and a cat, all dining together, each with their own plates, at a big square table in a field. That image made my spirit soar.

I stepped back and looked around, incredulous, at what destiny had manifested.

Epilogue

After the *Times* article appeared, hundreds of pet owners called me, desperate for someone to help their animals who were sick and dying after failed treatments at fancy, expensive hospitals in Manhattan. I transcribed each and every voice message into a brand-new, fat, spiral notebook with the date, owner's name and number, and medical problem of the animal.

One of the first things I discovered was that I was doing a disservice to my patients if I limited what was possible. Even though I'd had success helping dogs and cats to heal, for example, I didn't know what to do when people started calling with concerns about their unusual pets. I came to realize, however, that with God's help, the sky was the limit.

Rocky the Raccoon

I had been treating Julie's black Lab mix for arthritis for a few years but somehow I'd never met Rocky, the orphaned raccoon she'd rescued from her backyard and kept as a pet.

It took less time for me to review all I knew about raccoons—nothing—than it did for me to navigate the long, winding driveway leading to Julie's multimillion-dollar mansion.

Julie met me at the front door and led me to what she termed "Rocky's wing." The raccoon's elegant bedroom was tastefully furnished with family antiques. Julie hurried over to a large bureau and pulled open the middle drawer, "her favorite spot," Julie whispered. Inside lay a large raccoon. The jolt of the drawer must have disturbed her sleep, because Rocky lifted her sleepy head and peered out of the drawer at us with black beady eyes.

"Go ahead," Julie urged her sleepy pet. "Go say hello."

Riveted and wordless, I watched as Rocky's human-like hands grasped the edge of the drawer and heaved her body over and out of the drawer and onto the floor.

"I know, I know," Julie said, before I said anything. "She loves to eat, and she doesn't get enough exercise." The raccoon was nearly as big as Julie's lab.

Rocky hoisted herself up on the bed, and Julie told me to sit beside her. So I did. Rocky pushed her face right up to mine and pried my mouth open with her fingers. She pushed her snout into my mouth and sniffed. This unnerved me, to say the least, so I pulled back.

"Don't worry," Julie said, "this is the way she gets to know you."

Well, OK, I guess. I asked what was troubling Rocky.

"I have no idea why, but Rocky no longer uses her litter box."

Apparently, Julie had taught Rocky to use a litter box, just like a cat. But in recent weeks, the raccoon had been urinating on the furniture instead. Just as I wondered if excess weight might be making it difficult for her to climb into the box, Julie handed me a box of Rocky's favorite treat—organic corn cereal. "Feed her this," Julie told me. "That way she'll trust you and like you."

As I handed pieces of the cereal to the creature, which took them with her fingers and chewed delicately, I asked Julie to tell me a bit about Rocky's lifestyle. At night, the raccoon insisted on sleeping in bed with Julie and her husband, Jim, which relegated the cats and dogs to other parts of the house. Apparently, the various species didn't trust each other, so the dogs were gated in the kitchen and the cats were banished upstairs. Jim slept on the far end of the bed so Rocky could lay right next to Julie. Guests slept in the downstairs bedroom, because Rocky didn't like sharing the prime real estate upstairs.

As I continued to hand Rocky the cereal, I asked Julie if Rocky had any unusual likes or dislikes in the food department. This can be useful information when determining an appropriate homeopathic remedy. Julie couldn't think of any odd food choices but did note that the raccoon loved to drink.

"What kind of drinks are you talking about?" I asked.

"Well, you know, beer, wine, cocktails."

What? I imagined a formal cocktail party at the mansion, followed by a sit-down dinner, served by the butler, with the raccoon sitting among the other guests at the long mahogany dining room table. I mustered the courage to ask, "Do you offer her alcoholic beverages?"

"Of course not! It's just that we find her finishing all the drinks after a party when the guests have left."

I asked if Rocky's inappropriate urination started after one of these drinking binges. As with all problems, there's always a trigger. If my clients and I can figure out the causation, we are halfway to the solution.

The raccoon had been drinking for years, it turns out, but the peeing problem started about three weeks prior.

"Did anything unusual happen within the past six weeks?" Inciting factors tend to occur shortly prior to the dysfunction.

Julie stopped to think about it, then remembered that her conventional vet had administered a Rabies vaccine to Rocky about a week before the litter box issues began. *Aha!*

I examined the raccoon as best I could, but aside from her morbid obesity, Rocky seemed healthy. I left to work up her case at home on my computer. I promised to get back to Julie in a day or two.

Once back in my home office, I set to work on my homeopathic computer program. I highlighted "bad effects from the Rabies vaccine" and remembered to add an obscure rubric that Dr. Pitcairn had once mentioned, "forgetfulness of well-known streets." Given the timeline, I hypothesized that Rocky's Rabies shot had caused her to forget her toilet training.

Very few remedies turned up, but *Lachesis*, a common antidote to the bad effects of the Rabies vaccine, was one of them. I dissolved a few pellets of *Lachesis* in a one-ounce bottle of water and vodka (used to preserve the remedy). I felt it would be easier for Julie to administer it to the raccoon in a liquid state. Typically, I give owners the remedies in the form of a sweet-tasting powder, but in Rocky's case I thought it would be less stressful to squirt a little liquid into her mouth. Plus, Rocky might actually enjoy the vodka…

Three weeks later, Julie called for our follow-up. "First of all," she told me, "Rocky loved the medicine," (the vodka!) "and she's used the litter box each and every time!"

Then Julie added a postscript. "Not only that, but Rocky won't go near beer and wine anymore."

The news thrilled me, but I didn't understand why Rocky had become a teetotaler. I did some research and discovered that *Lachesis* can be a cure for alcoholism.

Alice the Bearded Dragon

One day, a woman called for an appointment for her bearded dragon, Alice. The worried woman told me that Alice hadn't eaten for a couple of weeks. I confessed to the woman that I'd never heard of bearded dragons so I was reluctant to take the case.

"I don't care," she said, "I have nowhere else to turn. I just spent thousands of dollars with the exotic pet specialist at the Animal Medical Center, and they couldn't figure out the problem."

I figured we had nothing to lose—plus, I was finding that homeopathy had helped many other animals that conventional medicine had deemed hopeless.

On the day of the appointment, Patricia, the owner, toted Alice into my Manhattan office in a large cat carrier. She put the bag on the exam table and carefully extracted a slender, horned creature, almost two-feet long. The creature just lay there.

Patricia's voice trembled as she told me that the pet specialist had drawn blood multiple times, X-rayed, and poked and prodded every orifice of the poor dragon, looking for answers. Finding none, she said, they recommended euthanasia as the "kindest option."

I eyed the poor critter as I began my homeopathic evaluation. I always start with focusing on the mental and emotional aspects of the patient. "Is she a needy lizard?" I asked Patricia. I felt ridiculous. "Is she friendly? Does she like company or is she independent?"

I, who prided myself on my ability to read animals' emotions, could not decipher any emotion as I looked into those cold reptilian eyes.

"Oh, she's so friendly!" Patricia exclaimed. "She loves company and affection."

I couldn't see it. The poor thing hadn't moved since it arrived. "How can you tell?" I asked, mystified.

"Well, she stays behind the couch all day while I am at work. The minute I come home she crawls out and gets up on the window ledge and looks out the window."

This was a trend. When Alice was happy she went to the window to sun herself and when no one was around she hid under the couch. *Who knew?* I continued my questioning. "What does she eat?" I didn't have a clue here.

"Crickets," she told me.

"Live ones?"

"Actually," Patricia said, "she used to eat live ones, but I recently switched to canned crickets. Actually, this whole problem started around that time."

Now we were getting somewhere. Perhaps she had eaten a bad cricket? Had this been a case of food poisoning? I'd had that a few times, and I was miserable. "Tell me, does she show any signs of abdominal discomfort?"

Patricia thought for a bit. "Maybe. Recently I found her on her back a few times when I came home from work. And she was scared, because she couldn't right herself."

This was beginning to make sense. Severe abdominal pain could have motivated Alice to flip on her back, thereby relieving the pressure—even though it is impossible for this type of lizard to right itself.

I continued. "How could you tell she was frightened?"

"Her color kept changing—she alternated from gray to white and her heart beat very fast."

Apparently she could feel the lizard's heart pulsing through its skin when they sat together watching TV.

My own heart was warming fast to this cold-blooded creature. I'd had no idea that reptiles shared the same emotions as we humans: loneliness, fear, and dare I even say, love?

I felt confident of my diagnosis. A bad cricket. I sent Alice home with one dose of *Nux Vomica*, a remedy useful for acute indigestion, which she was to administer when she got home.

The delighted owner called the next afternoon to report that Alice was her old self again. She'd eaten some crickets and spent the entire day on the window ledge basking in the sun.

Nugget the Hamster

Kellie brought her one-and-a-half-year-old hamster, Nugget, to my Greenwich Village office. He'd had difficulty walking recently, she said. I'd never had a hamster as a kid. My parents gave me the choice of a turtle or a bird. I had a painted turtle first, and, after he died, a parakeet named Blue Boy. Some of my friends had hamsters, gifts from their parents in lieu of a dog. A pet of last resort.

Before I started my homeopathic workup, I couldn't help myself. I had to ask, "Why did you choose a hamster for a pet?"

Kellie seemed surprised by my question. "There is no difference between a hamster and a dog. They are all family members," she said, adding, "I live in a studio, and I wanted a small-apartment companion."

I wouldn't have imagined that a hamster could provide the same depth of companionship as a dog.

Nugget was a very friendly, loving, and affectionate hamster, Kellie said. He licked her hand in affection as a dog or cat would. He knew his name, she said, and came when she called. He loved broccoli.

After Kellie cleaned his cage, he would race in.

She'd made a little cave for him out of a plastic can, and to Nugget this can in the cage was home sweet home, she said.

Nugget sounded like a happy little guy.

Then I learned that as much as Nugget loved his cage, if he saw that Kellie was leaving for an evening out, he would throw himself unhappily at the cage door.

I took the tiny little guy carefully in my hand, put him on his back and looked him over. I discovered a tumor the size of a marble in his armpit.

I knew that the remedy *Phosphorus* matched Nugget's emotional make-up: friendly, outgoing, affectionate, needs company. I'd also had success using *Phosphorus* in many cancer cases. I sent Kellie home with a dropper bottle of *Phosphorus* and instructed her to administer a few drops daily and to call me in a week.

At the follow-up call, Kellie told me that the tumor had shrunken to pea-sized and that Nugget was walking better every day. Interestingly, he was also urinating excessively, and although I didn't understand the mechanism, I surmised Nugget was eliminating the malignancy through the urine.

Both Kellie and I (and probably the hamster) were ecstatic.

Two months later, Kellie called again. Bad news. The tumor had regrown—bigger than ever. Mystified, I asked if anything unusual had occurred prior to the recurrence of the tumor. Kellie said she'd had to go away for two weeks on a work trip and left Nugget at home with a pet sitter. "Have you gone away much before?" I asked.

"Never more than a day."

I had seen many ailments exacerbate when owners left. I was pretty sure this was what had caused the regrown tumor. (Two weeks may not seem long to us but for hamsters it can seem like an eternity—the lifespan of a hamster is only two years.)

"How was Nugget when you returned?" I said.

"He was really mad at me when I got home," she said, adding that he took the sugar snap peas in his mouth and spit them at her. He had done this in the past, she said, but never to this degree. After throwing his entire meal at her, he nuzzled up to her and started cuddling. The poor guy. He'd missed her!

I sent Kellie home with *Staphysagria*, a remedy for suppressed anger and grief. The next morning, she called to report that Nugget was "super happy" to be with her. He cuddled nose to nose with her and no longer spat peas in her face.

The tumor had even begun to shrink!

A week later, Kellie called again. Nugget was acting strange, she said, and was storing his veggies "all over his litter." Fresh vegetables had been his favorite, she told me, preferring them to the pellets. Now he would only eat the pellets.

She told me that hamsters, like squirrels, naturally hoard their food, so they'll have a stash when food becomes irregular and sporadic. Although I knew next to nothing about hamsters, I knew a lot about abandonment and grief. I understood that Nugget was afraid that Kellie would leave him again, and in his mind, there would not be enough food (read love) for him. My heart broke for little Nugget. I put him back on the *Phosphorus*, and the tumor decreased for a short time, but his hoarding behavior escalated. Apparently, he never got over the grief. Still, Nugget managed to live out his entire two-year span on this earth.

Silvio the Flower Horn Fish

While at Sai Baba's ashram, I'd met a wonderful young couple, Michael and Alleli, who had started a residential school for abandoned, neglected, and abused children in a small village in India. After an evening with the couple and the thirty-four children, I told Michael that I would be honored to help in any way I could.

Back home, I received an email from Michael, telling me that Silvio, their flower horn fish, was desperately ill, his life floating in the balance. He had constant, mucousy diarrhea, was losing his color, and hadn't eaten in nine days. "He is usually a very hungry fish," Michael said.

I knew very little about fish (my final exam notwithstanding), but when I saw Silvio's picture on the email attachment, my heart melted. He was a large fish, nearly a foot long, and he was beautiful. His body was translucent white with various shades of purples, reds, and blues shimmering throughout. His cute fish face, with full puckered lips, practically begged to be kissed. He was the most adorable fish I had ever seen.

Michael had already consulted with the local veterinarians in India, as well as the aquarists, but to no avail. He was hoping I could refer a fish specialist in America. "I am comforted to know we have you to count on," Michael said.

I didn't know any fish specialists. And given my experience with conventional vet practices—I'd never seen anyone bring a fish into a hospital, except for lunch—I feared they might not have any more success than the Indian ones had. They'd suspected that Silvio had a bacterial infection in his intestine and had prescribed antibiotics. But after several rounds, Silvio seemed worse.

The veterinarians, aquarists, and Michael felt sure the key to the diagnosis and treatment lay in the type of mucous stool Silvio was excreting. I wasn't so sure. In the video Michael sent me of Silvio producing a bowel movement, I watched as the poor fish floated by, looking languid. He seemed sad.

I asked Michael if Silvio was a friendly fish. (Was I really asking this?) "Does he like people?"

"Oh yes, he loves the children, and the children love him," Michael said. He explained that when the school had acquired Silvio nine months before, they'd placed his big tank in the large room where the children lived and slept. "The kids play with him by trailing their fingers along the tank, and Silvio follows them back and forth."

Then I said, "Did anything in Silvio's life change prior to the onset of the diarrhea?"

Yes, in fact. The temperature in the village had soared, making it dangerous for the fish tank to remain in its usual place in the children's bedroom, Michael said, so they moved Silvio and his tank to a distant room with air conditioning. That's when the diarrhea started. In his new quarters, the caretaker had to change all of Silvio's water twice as often.

I sensed that Silvio felt lonely and isolated in his new air-conditioned room, too far for him to see and play with the kids.

There is one homeopathic remedy par excellence for acute recent grief: *Ignatia*. In fact, when *Ignatia* resolves a condition, it is evidence that grief is the etiology, or cause.

I instructed Michael to buy a strong potency of *Ignatia* and to pour some pellets into the tank. People and animals must dissolve the pellets in their mouth to be effective, but this seemed the only logical way to administer it to a fish.

I crossed my fingers and waited for the verdict.

The following day I sent an email. "How is Silvio? I love him and want him better!"

He wrote back. Silvio still had diarrhea "but looks not so bad."

Five days later I got an update. Silvio was looking brighter. "He is stable, responsive, and getting better and better daily" but he still hadn't eaten.

On the sixth day, I got another email. "He ate a guppy today!"

Bro the Golden Retriever

One beautiful summer day, Jo Ann breezed into my Connecticut office, supporting her Golden retriever's hind end with a makeshift harness, a towel on which she'd sewn handles.

Bro was thirteen and seemed healthy, but for the past six months he'd been paralyzed. It seems in the early spring he had become very weak, and eventually his back legs lost all capacity to move. Their veterinarian had no idea why this had occurred.

"He's perfect from the waist up," she said, smiling. "He's happy. My hope is to just make him more comfortable."

Bro seemed perfectly content lying on my yoga mat. I asked how she managed all eighty-five pounds of him.

"He doesn't know his back legs don't function," she insisted. "I had to learn 'the beat.'"

The beat?

"Each dog has its own beat. You just have to learn the beat," she said. "My feet become his back feet, so I have to learn the rhythm of his front feet. It is sort of like a horse with two clowns in the circus; one clown is the front of the 'horse' and the clown in the rear makes up the back feet. My feet are the back feet, and I move to the rhythm of his forelegs."

This reminded me of Phoebe, the paralyzed golden mix with a broken back.

"I need to keep his front legs working as if he has his hind legs, to give him confidence. It's like learning the cha-cha: back and forth, back and forth."

Going up the stairs proved challenging, but "we practiced a lot and once I got the beat it was a cinch." Same for getting in and out of the car—problem solved when she bought a second car, removed the passenger seat and put in a dog bed. Chuckling, she told me that she got pulled over by the cops constantly, as things didn't look right from the perspective of their patrol car.

A lot of old dogs become partially paralyzed due to degenerative disk disease. Handling them becomes such a burden that most owners opt for euthanasia, a decision they reach together with their veterinarians.

Jo Ann came to me because she had heard that acupuncture might make him more comfortable. I hoped for more, but I didn't feel optimistic after six months of complete hind-limb paralysis. Jo and Bro came three times a week for acupuncture. I didn't think it was working. But she said Bro was happier and was "trying to move his legs." I encouraged Jo Ann to switch modalities. In my experience, homeopathy was more powerful than acupuncture.

So many clients seek immediate, dramatic results. It was a delight to have a client feel otherwise, but I felt she was wasting her money, and I told her so. After several months I convinced her to give homeopathy a try. "We can always go back to acupuncture if homeopathy doesn't work," I told her.

My homeopathic workup led me to the remedy *Silicea*. I sent Jo Ann home with a dropper bottle and told her to call me in ten days.

Ten days later, she called.

"How is he doing?" I said. As usual, I had a pit in my stomach. I'm always anxious to know how the patient fared.

"Oh, he's a lot better, he's walking great."

Wait, what? I didn't believe her. She was so Pollyanna-ish that if Bro moved his legs just a little more while lying down, I believed she would say he was walking. "He's walking?"

"Yes, he's fine, he's walking great."

"Bring him right over, please."

One hour later, a 100 percent normal Bro walked into my front door. My mouth hung open in disbelief.

"I told you he was walking," Jo Ann said.

A few days after she'd started the *Silicea*, she realized she didn't have her purse so she dropped the support towel and ran to grab her purse. When she turned back, she saw Bro standing on his own. It happened to be Christmas morning, and he walked over to the Christmas tree.

"Faith," she told me, "a miracle dog."

Acknowledgments

First and foremost, I am forever grateful to Carol Dannhauser of the Fairfield County Writers' Studio, whose magical editing and steadfast support, especially during my darkest moments, made this book possible.

From the bottom of my heart, I thank Zoey O'Toole of Children's Health Defense, who championed my book, along with Louis Conte of Skyhorse Publishing. I am grateful to Caroline Russomanno for her prudent editing. A special thank you to Tony Lyons for taking a chance on me.

My heartfelt thanks to Louisa O'Neill, whose patience and support were invaluable.

Many thanks to Peter Hood for the beautiful cover photo of my dog Kyra, and for his dependable and constant support, which allowed me the time and the space to write my story.

Thank you to Dr. Sue Armstrong, VetMB, for her unfaltering support and belief in my book.

Profound appreciation for Dr. Richard Pitcairn, whose courage and integrity led to the resurgence of veterinary homeopathy in America and whose Professional Course started me on my life's work.

Special thanks to Dr. Jean Dodds for her courage and her determination to spread the truth throughout the world regarding vaccines and vaccine injury.

I'm grateful, especially, to two veterinarians, Dr. Larry Kahn and Dr. Henry Kellner, whose patience and kindness allowed me to blossom and to learn good conventional medicine.

Thank you to the many veterinary technicians who support and love their wards.

My friends Kim Ruska, Steven Warshawsky, Jessica DiDonato, Adele Ryan McDowell, Michelle Giancola, Rosemary Strauss, J.D. and Martha Brookshire, and many others read my book as I wrote. Their faith in me and my project helped me reach the finish line.

Lilliana, my spiritual "godmother," who took me under her wing at the ashram, and long after.

Thank you to Frank Caporale, whose generosity with his time and energy helped me pass the New York boards so many years ago.

Many thanks to Colette Griffin and Gy Davidson, for their unfaltering optimism and friendship over the decades.

Thanks to Toni Bradley, whose prayers undoubtedly reached their destination.

Thanks to my clients, who trusted me with their beloved pets, and to their animals that taught me so much.

A special thank you to my own dogs and cats, especially Shadow, Annie, Shanti, Tessa, Sienna, Destiny, Savannah, Kyra, Jyoti, and Zahara, for their unconditional love.

Thank you to the many angels in human form that God placed in my path.

I've been to Sai Baba's ashram twelve times. Each time, the ashram dogs remind me why I became a veterinarian.

I'm grateful for the many little miracles, including those disguised as disasters, that guided me on the journey to realize my soul purpose.

Ultimate thanks go to God, without Whom none of this would have been possible.